The
NHS
AT 70
A LIVING HISTORY

The
NHS
AT 70

A LIVING HISTORY

Ellen Welch

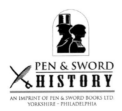

PEN & SWORD
HISTORY

AN IMPRINT OF PEN & SWORD BOOKS LTD.
YORKSHIRE - PHILADELPHIA

First published in Great Britain in 2018 by
PEN AND SWORD HISTORY
an imprint of
Pen & Sword Books Ltd
Yorkshire - Philadelphia

ISBN 978 1 52671 737 5

A CIP catalogue record for this book is available from the British Library.

Typeset in Sabon 11/13.5 By
Aura Technology and Software Services, India
Printed and bound in England
by CPI Group (UK) Ltd, Croydon, CR0 4YY.

Pen & Sword Books Ltd incorporates the Imprints of Pen & Sword Books
Archaeology, Atlas, Aviation, Battleground, Discovery, Family History, History,
Maritime, Military, Naval, Politics, Railways, Select, Transport, True Crime,
Fiction, Frontline Books, Leo Cooper, Praetorian Press, Seaforth Publishing,
Wharncliffe and White Owl.

For a complete list of Pen & Sword titles please contact

PEN & SWORD BOOKS LIMITED
47 Church Street, Barnsley, South Yorkshire, S70 2AS, England
E-mail: enquiries@pen-and-sword.co.uk
Website: www.pen-and-sword.co.uk

or

PEN AND SWORD BOOKS
1950 Lawrence Rd, Havertown, PA 19083, USA
E-mail: Uspen-and-sword@casematepublishers.com

Contents

Acknowledgements

When I agreed to write a book on the history of the NHS in time for the 70th birthday celebrations, I hadn't really appreciated the scale of the project I had taken on. Encapsulating an institution which has undergone so many changes, and presenting it as something readable, was an overwhelming prospect, and since the NHS has been described as the closest thing the English people have to a religion, I felt a weight of responsibility to do it justice and I have a lot of people to thank for helping me finish it.

The personal accounts are what bring this book to life. All of us in the UK have an NHS story to tell, and I would have liked to fill the pages with many more. I am indebted to all of the contributors, who took the time to write their accounts - a massive thank you for your efforts to Noreen and Janyce Quigley, Rose Singleton, Kate Cavanagh, Meg Parkes, Geoff Gill, Judith Susser, David Wingfield, Lianna Brinded, Hannah Ramsdale, Alison Gill, Neil Barnard, Irina Bardsley and Carol Trow.

As a declaration of interests, I am a doctor, and I have worked in both public and private healthcare settings in the UK, in New Zealand and as a cruise ship doctor in an American system. The views in this book are my own. I am by no means an 'NHS expert' and in fact I learnt a lot about the NHS during my research for this book. In the further reading section, I point you towards the texts of many more learned people who have spent years writing about the NHS and health policy, and whose work helped to shape this book. I have attempted to transform the history of the NHS into a digestible book that can be understood. All facts and figures are from references sources, which have not been highlighted in the text to make it an easier read, but can be found at the back of the book, and I am happy to have any inaccuracies corrected.

Carol and Laura and the team at Pen & Sword worked very hard to ensure the book was finished on time when I had overrun my deadlines, and helped to bring the final product together - thank you for your patience. Thank you to those who provided images, and took the time to help. Thanks to my ship family for being patient with me always running off to write, and to my actual family, especially Nikola, for the support. Most of all, thank you to Kate, who was my biggest cheerleader during this project and helped me every step of the way, with contributing, proof reading and encouraging me to continue.

Preface

'Medical treatment should be made available to rich and poor alike in accordance with medical need and no other criteria. The essence of a satisfactory health service is that the rich and poor are treated alike. Poverty is not a disability and wealth is not an advantage.'

Aneurin Bevan – Health Secretary 1946

At midnight on 5 July 1948, the National Health Service was born, with the founding principle to be free at the point of use and based on clinical need rather than on a person's ability to pay. Seventy years since its formation, these core principals still hold true, although the world we now live in is a very different place to the post-war era in which it was formed, and the long-term sustainability of the service in its current form is questionable.

Broken from two world wars, undernourished with rationing still in place, and relying on a bucket in front of the fire for the weekly wash – the average life expectancy in 1948 was 60 years old. A child born in 2018 can expect to live to an average age of 80. Over the last century, infant mortality rates have fallen dramatically as standards of living have improved, with rates 30 times lower at the end of the twentieth century than at the start. Immunisation has virtually eliminated death from infectious diseases such as measles, mumps, rubella, poliomyelitis, diphtheria, tetanus and whooping cough. In 1901, the majority of people died young – only 25 per cent of deaths occurred in people over the age of 65; a century later, this had risen to 80 per cent. Deaths due to cardiovascular disease have declined as lifestyles have become healthier, while deaths from cancers have increased, as we are living longer (5 per cent of deaths were from cancers in 1901 compared to 25 per cent in 2000).

The twentieth century was rife with innovation. The discovery of DNA in the 1950s helped to revolutionize the future prevention and treatment of many diseases. Organ transplants, now a commonplace procedure, were pioneered in the 1960s, and milestones in women's rights and fertility were achieved with the legalisation of abortion and improved accessibility to the contraceptive pill. The 1970s saw the introduction of CTs, MRI scanners and 'test tube babies' and in the 1980s, cancer treatments improved and breast screening was introduced. We now have expert patients and health charities, and a very different GP waiting room to the one of 1948.

The NHS is the largest and oldest publicly funded healthcare system in the world and provides anyone registered with an NHS number with medical care, without a medical bill at the end of the consultation. It is funded chiefly from taxation and National Insurance contributions. In the early 1950s, charges were introduced for dental services, prescriptions and spectacles (prompting Bevan to resign from cabinet in protest). Today, as we live longer, demand for services continues to grow, and the NHS budget gets stretched thinner and thinner, it has been suggested that people start paying for other NHS services such as routine appointments to see their GP. The slow privatisation of the NHS is moving away from the core values that it was founded upon. Are these values idealistic and unsustainable in modern Britain? Danny Boyle's 2012 Olympic Games opening ceremony brought a tear to many an eye, celebrating the NHS as 'the institution which more than any other unites our nation'. It is not sustainable in its current form. To avoid a move to the American system, where people are bankrupted for medical care, or resort to 'go fund me' pages to raise money to pay for that emergency surgery for a burst appendix, to avoid a similar system emerging in the UK then something does need to change. Less political involvement – the NHS should not be something that wins election votes. Health policies need to be evidence based and sustainable, and not formulated to win the next election.

This book attempts to summarise the foundations of the NHS and discuss why it was formed, provide an understanding of its current structure and problems and consider what the future may hold.

Chapter 1

Pre-NHS Britain

Organised health care really started to take shape in the nineteenth century, but clearly medicine and healthcare have been around a whole lot longer than this. Whole libraries are dedicated to the history of medicine, and this chapter is in no way comprehensive, but aims to present a snapshot of healthcare and medicine over the last few centuries, to gain a flavour of what Britain was like, and to appreciate how life has evolved into the system we know today.

The Middle Ages (500-1500) and
The Renaissance (1400-1700)

Medieval medics were pretty powerless in the face of disease, and medical knowledge and ideas about treatments were often based on superstition. The cause of disease was considered supernatural, and herbal remedies were commonplace.

Responsibility for the poor, sick and elderly traditionally fell to the church, and prior to the development of hospitals, townsfolk would turn to their nearest monastery for help with their sick. Prayer rituals were used to heal, and monks produced some of the earliest medical texts documenting the herbal mixtures they used to return their patients back to good health. Religious men were forbidden to spill blood (by Papal decree), so it was common at the time for barbers to assist monks in procedures considered dirty and beneath them – such as bloodletting and leeching, extracting teeth, lancing boils and doing a quick short back and sides (Box 1.1)

Barber Surgeons

Left: A barber-surgeon extracting stones from a woman's head; symbolising the expulsion of 'folly' (insanity). Watercolour by J. Cats, 1787, after B. Maton. (Wellcome Collection)

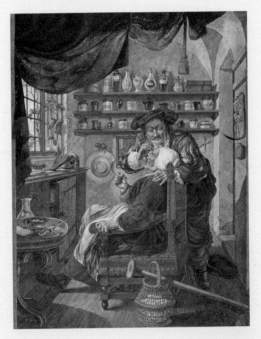

Below: High Street of Edinburgh in the 18th century – Note the barber-surgeon's pole with bleeding bowl on the left. Lithograph by W and A K Johnston, 1852 (M McLaren, The Capital Of Scotland, Edinburgh 1950) (via Wikimedia Commons)

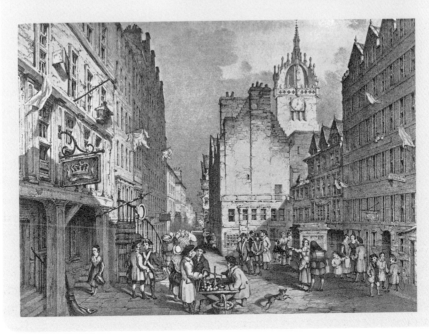

For centuries, surgery was a craft carried out by barbers, and early versions of the Hippocratic Oath actually cautioned physicians from practicing surgery. Medieval barbers provided their patients with analgesia using substances such as opium, mandrake root, and hemlock, and, if they didn't pass away due to intoxication, surgery could be performed using wine to clean the wounds. Minor procedures and teeth pulling were commonplace, but internal surgery was also attempted, such as removal of bladder stones, castration of local rapists, and trephining the skulls of epileptic patients to allow the demons to escape. Bloodletting was one of their key duties. It was believed that draining away blood would also drain away the disease. Physicians still considered themselves the 'real doctors' and even when hospitals were established, the barbers did not have a place there, and typically practiced in marketplaces, advertising their business with the familiar red and white striped pole – still seen outside modern hairdressers today – which represented blood and bandages.

As universities developed during the Renaissance, anatomy and surgery began to be studied in more detail. A split formed between academically trained surgeons, who wore long robes, and the 'trained on the job' barber surgeons, who wore shorter robes. In 1540, barbers and surgeons joined forces to gain credibility for their trade and formed the Company of Barber Surgeons. The invention of gunpowder led to new injuries during warfare and barber surgeons such as Frenchman Ambroise Paré made headlines for his work inventing surgical instruments and improving surgical treatments. The advent of anaesthesia and aseptic techniques improved complication and infection rates and as more patients benefited, surgeons gained greater respect. Gradually, due to pressure from the medical profession to distinguish themselves from lesser esteemed back street barbers, surgeons split away from the Company of Barbers to form the Royal College of Surgeons in 1800 and began to hold exams for membership. Prior to this, surgeons were not legally permitted to prescribe internal medicines for their patients – this was a privilege reserved for the learned physicians, who had earned their doctorates of medicine at University. One tradition that still persists to this day is the use of the title 'Mr' or 'Miss' instead of 'Dr' when surgeons qualify as a Member of the Royal College of Surgeons, as a nod to their roots. All surgeons clearly now have to pass a medical degree prior to their years of training in surgery, and they are no longer required to perform haircuts.

In the late 1530s, there were nearly 900 religious houses in England, whose primary function was to provide lodging for travellers and pilgrims, and to act as almshouses and schools. They typically imposed local taxes to assist them in providing such charity. Following the Dissolution of the Monasteries (1536-1540) by Henry VIII, almost all of these institutions were disbanded, creating considerable hardship for the poor and destitute who were thrown out onto the street. Only three London hospitals survived the dissolution, after the citizens of the city petitioned for them to remain – St Barthlolomew's (Bart's), St Thomas's and St Mary's of Bethlehem. They were endowed by the king himself, as the first example of secular support being provided for medical institutions. They remained the principal hospitals in the country until the voluntary hospital movement began in the nineteenth century.

The Renaissance was a period of discovery in medicine. The scientific method was established, and universities established schools of medicine. Artists such as Da Vinci revolutionized painting, and dissection allowed the human body to be studied in more detail, which improved knowledge of anatomy. The invention of the printing press allowed ideas to be disseminated more quickly around Europe, allowing knowledge to be shared. In the 1620s, William Harvey showed that blood circulates, challenging Galen's theory of humours (that disease was due to an imbalance of the four humours – blood, phlegm, black bile and yellow bile) which had been fundamental for centuries – and queried the need for the well-established practice of bloodletting.

Outbreaks of infection still defied medical knowledge. The Black Plague rampaged through Europe in the fourteenth century, recurring in outbreaks until the nineteenth century, claiming over 200 million lives. People believed the pandemic was a punishment from God, and blame was dispensed indiscriminately to groups deemed responsible – such as beggars, lepers, Jews and pilgrims. Individuals with skins diseases such as acne or psoriasis were exterminated, and religious fanaticism bloomed. 'Cures' for the plague included pressing a plucked chicken against the plague sores; smoking tobacco (a novel new substance recently introduced from the New World); use of posies and perfumes; dried toad; leeches; a lucky hares foot ... We now know that plague can be successfully treated with antibiotics, but these, along with public health measures, had not yet been discovered.

Modern History

Improvements in public health and understanding of infection began to develop in the 1800s. In 1796, Edward Jenner discovered vaccinations, by famously using cowpox to protect against smallpox, and some 60 years later, Louis Pasteur developed germ theory, which proved a link between dirt and disease.

The Industrial Revolution resulted in more families moving to towns and cities, often sharing squalid, overcrowded accommodation, and standards of public health were poor. Pollution, contaminated water and a limited diet allowed infectious diseases to flourish and cholera epidemics were commonplace. An increased understanding of disease and hygiene led to improvements in public health standards. In 1854, John Snow showed the source of the London cholera epidemic to be the communal water pump used at Broad Street. Edwin Chadwick was a social reformer, who worked with the Poor Law Commission. He raised awareness that dirt and squalor are associated with high mortality rates, and that the misery faced by the poor was something the government could control, and not due to some innate shortcoming of the working class. His work led to the first Public Health Act in Britain in 1848, 100 years prior to the creation of the NHS, which led to improvements in the sewage system and building regulations, which contributed to declining mortality rates.

During the nineteenth and early twentieth centuries, great advances were seen in medicine and public health. Anaesthesia and aseptic surgery were introduced; game changing discoveries were made – such as penicillin, x-rays and radium, and blood groups which enabled blood transfusion. The two world wars shaped medicine, and the injuries caused by the heavy artillery of the First World War meant that medicine was forced to pioneer new techniques in plastic surgery and skin grafting, and develop specialities such as maxillofacial surgery. Rationing improved the diets of some and encouraged healthy eating. Events during the Second World War created the stage for the formation of the NHS. Social barriers were broken down and brought people together, looking for improvements in society – more about this in chapter 2.

Workhouses and the Poor Law

The history of the workhouse as an institution to solve the enduring problem of poverty spans over three centuries and was an important

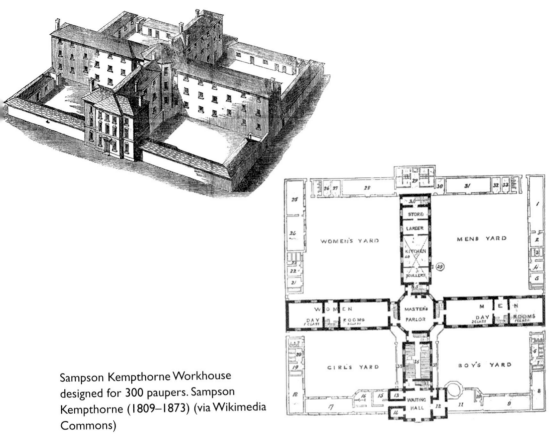

Sampson Kempthorne Workhouse designed for 300 paupers. Sampson Kempthorne (1809–1873) (via Wikimedia Commons)

There is a key that accompanies this image if there is room:

1. Work Room
2. Store
3. Receiving Wards, 3 beds
4. Bath
5. Washing Room
6. Receiving Ward, 3 beds
7. Washing Room
8. Work Room
9. Flour and Mill Room
10. Coals
11. Bakehouse
12. Bread Room
13. Searching Room
14. Porter's Room
15. Store
16. Potatoes
17. Coals
18. Work Room
19. Washing Room
20. Receiving Ward, 3 beds
21. Washing Room
22. Bath
23. Receiving Ward, 3 beds
24. Laundry
25. Wash-house
26. Dead House
27. Refractory Ward
28. Work Room
29. Piggery
30. Slaughter House
31. Work Room
32. Refractory Ward
33. Dead House
34. Women's Stairs to Dining Hall
35. Men's Stairs to ditto
36. Boys' and Girls' School and Dining Room
37. Delivery
38. Passage
39. Well
40. Cellar under ground

RULES AND ORDERS

To be observed by every Person belonging to the
WORK-HOUSE *of the Parish of St. John, at* **HACKNEY,**
In the County of **MIDDLESEX.**

That before an Order is made for the Admission of any Person into the House, that an Inventory be taken by the Churchwarden, or some Person deputed by him, of what Household Goods and Clothes they are possessed of; and after an Order is made for their Admission, that they be delivered up to the Mistress, in order to be cleaned and made useful for the Service of the House; and that they be new clothed, if thought necessary by the Committee, and have their proper Apartments and Employments assigned them by the Committee appointed to manage the House. And if any Person shall conceal any Linnen, or Woollen, belonging to the House, with an Intent to steal or imbezzle the same, such Person shall immediately be carried before a Magistrate, in order to be imprisoned and punished with the utmost Rigour as the Law directs.

II. THAT Prayers be read in this House every Morning by the Mistress, or some Person deputed by her, before Breakfast; and every Evening before Supper; and that Grace be Said before, and Thanks returned after, each Meal; and all those that are able, and do not attend Prayers, to lose their next Dinner.

III. ALL that are able, and in Health, to go every *Sunday* to Church, or some other Place of Religious Worship, Morning and Afternoon : That they return Home as soon as Divine Service is over; and if any be found loitering, or begging by the Way, to lose their next Meal. If, at any Time, they get drunk, or are guilty of prophane Cursing or Swearing, to be punished in the Stocks as the Law directs.

IV. THAT no Person be permitted to go out of the House without Leave from the Committee, unless upon some great Emergency; and that, in such Case, one of the Churchwardens, or Overseers of the Poor, or one of the Committee in waiting, is desired to give Leave, if they find it necessary; and if they do not return within the Time allowed them, that the Mistress do not presume to let them into the House again without the Consent of the Committee.

V. THAT no distilled Liquors be brought into the House without Leave from the Committee, nor any strong Beer without Leave from the Mistress; and whoever shall disturb the House by brawling, quarrelling, fighting, or abusive Language, shall lose one Day's Meal, and for the second Offence be put into the dark Room twenty four Hours.

VI. THAT every Person in Health shall be kept to such Labour as they can well do, according to their several Ages and Abilities; that is to say, from *Lady-day* to *Michaelmas*, from Six of the Clock in the Morning to Six at Night; from *Michaelmas* to *Lady-day*, from Seven in the Morning till Five at Night (Meal-time excepted); and if any grown Person refuse to work, to be kept on Bread and Water, or expell'd the House : The Children to be corrected by the Mistress.

VII. THAT all Persons, who through Idleness may pretend themselves Sick, Lame, or Infirm, so as to be excused their Working; such Impostors so discovered either by their Stomachs or the Apothecary, shall be carried before a Magistrate, in order to be punished as the Law directs.

VIII. THAT a Bell be rung every Morning, in the Summer, from *Lady-day* to *Michaelmas* by Five, and from *Michaelmas* to *Lady-day* by Six, for the healthful People to rise to work. and to go to Bed in the Summer by Nine, and in the Winter by Eight : and that the Mistress see all the Candles out at those Times.

IX. THAT all the Beds be made in the Morning by Nine, and every Room and Passage swept and cleaned by Ten; to be washed as often as the Occasion shall require, and the windows let open at all convenient Times to air the Rooms; the Dishes to be washed twice a Day, or oftner; no waste to Fire to be made, and in the Summer none at all, except in the Infirmary-Kitchen, and Wash-house in the Time of Washing and Ironing.

X. THAT all the Children be washed, combed and cleaned by Eight in the Morning, and some proper Persons chose to teach them to read; and that they be taught to labour and work, as the Committee shall direct, in such Manufactures as may be most useful and beneficial for the publick Good, and not permitted to play till they have finished their Tasks.

XI. THAT all Provisions be cleanly and well dressed; to go to Breakfast in Summer at Eight, in the Winter at Nine, Dinner all the Year at One, Supper in the Evening at Six; to be allowed half an Hour at Breakfast, and a whole Hour at Dinner; and all that have not done their Talk by Supper, to work afterwards until finished : And that great Care be taken that they fit decently at Meal, and that the Bell be rung to call them to their Meals.

XII. THAT the Nurses take Care to make and mend all the Linnen and Clothes When any Person dies, to deliver his or her Clothes clean and neat to the Mistress, to be laid up in the Ward-Robe or Store-Room, and also every Thing else they die possessed of, for the Use the House.

XIII. THAT if any Person fall sick or lame, Notice thereof to be given by the Mistress to the Apothecary or Surgeon with all convenient Speed, to be taken Care of; and such other Victuals than what is daily used, be allowed the Patient, as shall be thought proper by the Apothecary or Surgeon, or either of them.

XIV. THAT no Person be allowed to any Person out-of the House, unless in cases of Lunacy, Plague, Small-pox, Foul-disease, or Idiotism; and that all the Money received or collected for the use of the Poor of this Parish, (Sacrament-Money excepted) shall be brought to Account, and applied to the Support of this House, and the Maintenance of the Poor therein, and not otherwise appropriated.

XV. THAT no Person of either Sex be allowed to smoke in Bed, or in any Bed-chamber of the House.

XVI. THAT a Book be kept, wherein the Christian and Sur-names of every grown Person shall be set down, and called over every Morning by Six in the Summer, and by Eight in the Winter, and at One in the Afternoon; and if any of the said Persons are missing, or any other Offences committed by any Persons in the House, the same shall be noted and set down, in order that the Offender may be examined by the Committee, and brought to such Punishment as the Nature of the Offence shall require.

XVII. THAT Two of the Committee, with one of the Churchwardens, or Overseers of the Poor, do meet at the Work-house once in every Week at least, to examine all the Provisions that are brought into the House, with the Prices and Quantity, and enter them into a Book, to be kept for that Purpose; and to see that each person hath the following Allowance and no more; and to examine into the Management of the Mistress; and likewise to hear and examine into the Complaints and Grievances of the Poor, (if any) and report to the next General Meeting:

To wit.   7 Ounces of Meat when dressed, without   }
            Bones, to every grown Person,
            2 Ounces of Butter,   }
            4 Ounces of Cheese,   } Every day
            1 Pound of Bread,   }
            3 Pints of Beer,   }
            The Children at the Discretion of the
            Mistress.

XVIII. THAT every person do endeavour to preserve a good Unity, and look upon themselves as one family. And to prevent any Dispute which may create Differences amongst themselves, by forging and telling Lies, such Persons so offending (on good Proof to the Committee) shall be set on a Stool in the most publick Place in the Dining-Room, whilst the Family are at Dinner, and a Paper fixed on his or her Breast with these Words wrote, *Infamous Lyar*; and likewise to lose that Meal.

XIX. THAT Care be taken that none of the Materials of the several Manufactures be wasted or spoiled; That there be no defacing of Walls, or breaking of Windows; And that these Orders be publickly read once every Week, that none may plead or pretend Ignorance.

XX. THAT the Committee in waiting do order the Grand Committee to be summoned as Occasion shall require.

XXI. THAT for the Future, if any Person shall apply to be put into the Work-house, that he, she, or they, be referred to the Committee at their Weekly Meeting next after any such Application; and that the Churchwardens and Overseers of the Poor, do make proper Provision for such Person or Persons, 'till such Meeting, as the Necessity of the Case shall require; and that neither they, nor any of them, do send any Person or Persons into the Work-house in the Interval of such Meetings, unless in some extraordinary Case, occasioned by Sickness or Accident.

Workhouse Rules at the Hackney Workhouse 1750 Taken from The Workhouse Website: http://www.workhouses.org.uk/Hackney/index. shtml#rules

precursor to the NHS. During the reign of Elizabeth I, in 1601, the Act for the Relief of the Poor (which is now known as the Old Poor Law) was passed to deal with beggars, who were viewed as a threat to civil order. This Act made local parishes responsible for the poor and decreed that the 'impotent poor' – the old and sick – were to be cared for in poorhouses, while able bodied paupers should be given work and sent to prison if they refused. Individual parishes were responsible for overseeing their own areas, and at its inception, local populations were small enough for communities to be aware of each other's circumstances, meaning the 'idle poor' were unable to abuse the system. Relief under the 'Old Poor Law' was either in the form of 'indoor relief' – assistance inside a workhouse or almshouse – or 'outdoor relief', which involved payment in the form of money, food, blankets or clothing. Funding to provide this assistance was collected by Overseers of the Poor, who levied local property owners (a tax that we still pay today now, known as council tax).

There was no uniformity to the system throughout the country, and many paupers migrated towards the more generous parishes. During the seventeenth century, the workhouses evolved as a way of allowing parishes to avoid outdoor relief payments. By 1776, in London alone, over 16,000 people were housed in one of the city's eighty workhouses – which amounted to 1-2 per cent per cent of the capital's population. There was rumbling dissatisfaction with this system, and its critics considered the conditions in many of these 'Paupers Palaces' to be too comfortable, encouraging idleness and pauperism. The New Poor Law was therefore passed in 1834, to cut expenditure and abolish pauperism by attempting to ensure only the truly destitute would accept poor relief. Those eligible could not be better off than the worst paid independent worker, and if they were truly needy, they would be offered the workhouse – a harsh and austere regimen which only the desperate would enter willingly. It was not a prison, and people could come and go if they found work, but the regime was strict (see Box 1.5 – workhouse rules) and to go into the workhouse was considered the ultimate degradation. Poverty was considered to be a moral failing rather than a misfortune. Inmates' heads were shaved and they were given rough, uncomfortable workhouse uniforms to wear. They engaged in manual labour such as stone breaking and rope picking. Food provided was basic and monotonous such as gruel (watery porridge – Oliver Twist style), broth, bread and beer (safer than water). Orphaned children would be housed alongside unmarried mothers, the elderly, and the mentally and physically ill – conditions were overcrowded and dirty. Families were separated and parents had restricted contact with their children, often only seeing them once a week for a few hours. Many workhouses had designated wards or annexes for sick paupers, and the nursing care was often carried out by other inmates. Paid nursing, during this period, was considered a job for poor, elderly women and was associated with drunkenness, bad language and a casual attitude to patients. Workhouse unions at the time were required to appoint a medical officer, who was usually part time and poorly paid. Joseph Rogers wrote his memoirs about his time as the workhouse doctor at the Strand Union Workhouse. He reported that he had no qualified nurses to care for over 500 sick inmates. If he wished to administer medication, the bill for this would come out of his pay of £50 a year, meaning that treating patients prevented him from making a living.

He described workhouse doctors who routinely gave coloured water for every ailment to avoid medication charges.

Standards continued to be poor until concerns were raised in the 1860s. Prominent figures of the day such as Florence Nightingale commented that these hospitals were as bad, or worse than the military hospitals she had encountered during the Crimean war (1853-1856). In 1865, medical journal the *Lancet* investigated conditions in workhouse infirmaries and produced scathing reports, which prompted the government to conduct their own inquiries. Inspectors found poorly ventilated wards with no washing facilities. They found infectious fever patients scattered through the wards to infect other inmates. 'Lunatics' shared wards with no medical supervision. The only paid nurse employed at the Rotherhithe workhouse infirmary, Matilda Beeton, also spoke of her experiences, reporting that untrained pauper nurses beat the patients and stole their food. She reported dirty patients, crawling with vermin and sleeping in maggot infested beds, and 'an insufficiency of everything', complaining that the same towels used for wiping down patients were used as teacloths. 'It did not seem to me,' said Beeton, 'that a pauper's life was regarded in any other light than the sooner they were dead the better.'

By the end of the nineteenth century, parliament passed the Metropolitan Poor Act, to improve these appalling conditions, which authorized the building of separate workhouse infirmaries, with trained medical and nursing staff. Nightingale and her contemporaries helped to change the attitudes of the day, setting up organized training schools and emphasizing the need for properly trained nurses in all hospitals.

In addition to these poor law institutes, local authorities (the Metropolitan Asylums Board) set up institutions which could be accessed by the entire population, not just the poor. Hospitals were built specifically to care for fever patients – those suffering from infectious diseases such as smallpox and tuberculosis – and asylums for the mentally ill. This publicly owned system of hospitals was effectively the foundation for what became the NHS in 1948. This process started in 1929, when a further Act of Parliament transferred the powers and responsibilities of the Poor Law to local government authorities, who took over the administration of the poor law infirmaries, as well as the fever hospitals and asylums.

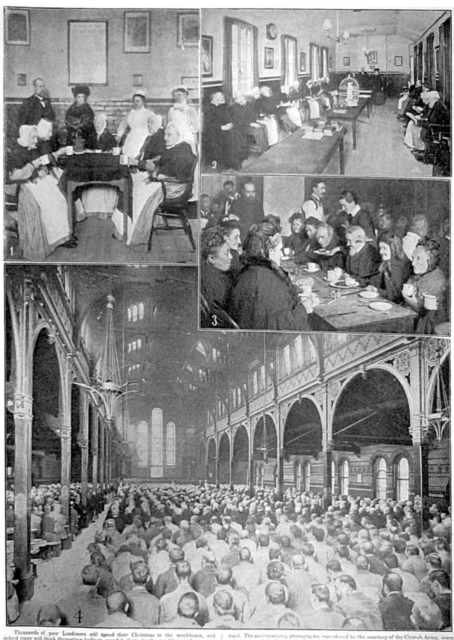

Winter in the Workhouse The *Graphic*, 21 December 1907 (unknown author via Wikimedia Commons)

Florence Nightingale (1820-1910)

Florence Nightingale was a celebrated British nurse and the founder of modern nursing. She became famed as the 'Lady with the Lamp' during the Crimean War, when she took a team of nurses out to improve the conditions and cleanliness in the military hospitals. Nightingale was a believer in the miasma theory, that disease was spread through foul air, and pointed out that more troops died from diseases such as cholera, typhoid and dysentery than from their battle wounds, and she campaigned for improved sanitation. Her nightly rounds with her lamp, checking on the soldiers gained their respect and she returned to Britain a heroine. Donations poured into her 'Nightingale fund' which she used to establish the Nightingale Training School at St Thomas's Hospital in London, which transformed nursing from a lowly, unwholesome job, to a professional career, teaching nurses discipline and practical skills. She pioneered infection control measures and influenced ward designs, realizing that the setup of a hospital can affect the health and recovery of its patients, and the classic 'Nightingale wards' as shown on page 24 bear her name.

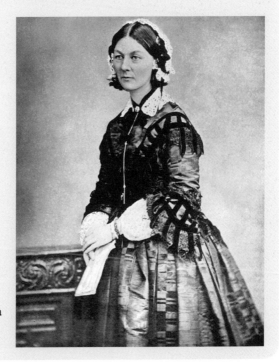

Florence Nightingale circa 1860. (via Wikimedia Commons)

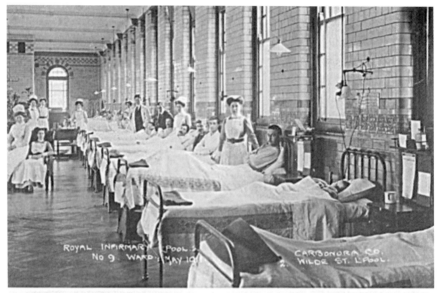

NO. 9 WARD, ROYAL INFIRMARY, LIVERPOOL, May 1911

Nightingale ward 1911– Royal Liverpool Infirmary (Used with permission from The Liverpool Nurses League)

Voluntary Hospitals

In stark contrast to these municipal or public hospitals were the Voluntary hospitals. 'Voluntaries' as they were known, were funded by the voluntary contributions of investors and philanthropists. Many had been founded centuries before and they included most of London's best-known teaching hospitals and some smaller cottage hospitals run by GPs in more rural areas. Some, like Bart's, claimed a medieval origin, while many more were formed in the early eighteenth century, such as the Edinburgh Royal Infirmary, the Bristol Royal Infirmary and Addenbrookes in Cambridge. Voluntary hospitals were autonomous and could choose not only who they wanted to employ, but who they wanted to treat. Charitable donations were dependent on high cure rates, meaning that elderly patients and those with chronic disease were unlikely to be admitted. The voluntary hospitals were renowned for cutting edge medicine and medical education, and in 1834, the Select Committee on Medical education commented that these voluntary hospitals were a major source of the advancement of medical science. The voluntary hospitals had strict admission criteria, requiring either a letter of recommendation from a hospital governor or subscriber, or the payment of fees. The payment of fees was variable – some were paid by family and friends or by the parish; while others prepared for being sick, by making weekly payments to a hospital contributory scheme. All patients were required to provide financial security to cover burial costs if they died in hospital. In some cases, hospitals would waive fees, in cases of extreme need. Many hospitals would reject patients suffering with venereal disease, and hospitals such as St Thomas's, that did accept them, housed them in designated 'foul wards' and upped their fees (10s 6d versus 3s 6d in the late eighteenth century). Hospital patients tended to come from the lower classes, as the wealthy preferred to pay doctors to treat them in their own homes.

In the 1890s, the voluntary hospitals ran alongside the local government and poor law hospitals, providing approximately 26 per cent per cent of the nation's beds, leaving the majority of the chronically unwell and psychiatric cases to the other institutes. This figure rose to 33 per cent per cent in 1938. As medicine advanced and there was a focus on teaching and research, doctors (and governors) in voluntary hospitals became even more selective of their patients, choosing those with diseases of interest, or of a short term nature to ensure a rapid turnover of patients. This rigid system led the way for the expansion of the old workhouse or public hospitals to fill the gaps. By the 1920s, many of these 'workhouse infirmaries' were larger than the old workhouses themselves. Many had resident medical staff and facilities for x-rays, laboratory tests and surgery. It became customary for the voluntaries to transfer their 'unwanted cases' such as cancer patients, or those with infectious disease, to the local authority hospitals.

Through the 1930s and 1940s, pressure for reform of the health services grew. Charity donations, which the voluntaries depended on, declined, and the emergency response coordinated by the government during wartime – which involved all the hospitals working together to share staff and resources, demonstrated how a universal system may work. Bevan's NHS Act's brought the voluntary hospitals into public ownership, and from then on, they were funded from general taxation, staffed by salaried consultants and professional administrators.

My NHS Story

Noreen Quigley is a retired nurse from County Durham who completed her training at the dawn of the NHS. (Oral history taken by her daughter Janyce Quigley)

'I started my nurse training aged 17 as a "pre-probationer" in 1946 at Holmside and South Moor Hospital, which was a cottage hospital with about 48 beds for miners and their families. When I was 18, I moved to Sunderland General Hospital where I trained as a State Registered Nurse (SRN) for 3 years and in those days, you lived at the hospital where you trained. You had to be back in the nurse's home, signed in on a register by 10pm at night – I won't tell you the number of times I slipped down the fire escape to go to a Dance! As soon as I finished, I received a letter from the Matron back at the miner's hospital offering

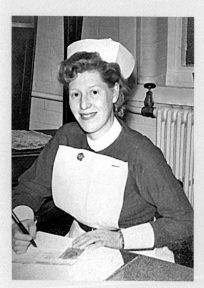
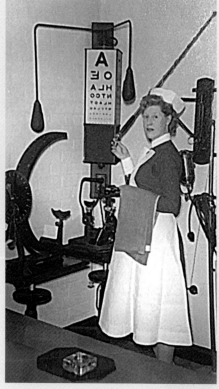

Noreen Quigley 1950 (2 images)

me a position as night sister and I was amazed to be told I could live at home. I returned there when I was 21, in 1950, and it was no longer a miner's hospital, but an NHS hospital.

'I loved being a nurse. You really had to want to do the job back then, as the times were difficult, and it was hard physical work, but I liked it a lot. Nursing seems different now, and when I visit hospitals, all I seem to see is nurses writing. I was a night sister for general surgery and medicine. We worked 12-hour shifts starting at 20:15 until 0815 the following day. We checked pressure points twice a day. Matron did her rounds every morning, and woe betide us if she found even a speck of dust during her inspections. We had side wards for the sickest patients, but these were also used for private patients. We looked after them the same as the NHS patients, but the surgeon would be the one who benefited. I never agreed with having private patients in an NHS hospital.'

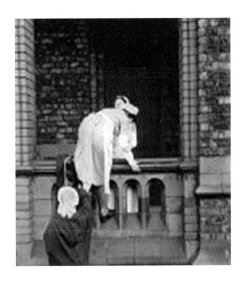

Late for Duty
(Liverpool Nurses League)

The Dispensaries

Dispensaries formed a key part of healthcare for several hundred years, before they were absorbed into the NHS in 1948, and then largely forgotten. They were charitable organisations, where medical advice and medications could be dispensed – generally for free, or for a minimal fee, and if patients could afford to pay for a doctor, then they were not supposed to make use of the dispensaries. They ran on a subscriber system, similar to that used in the Voluntary hospitals, which relied on the funding of rich philanthropists, who would select patients from the 'deserving poor' to use the services they had sponsored. They would introduce the patient to the dispensary by handing over a note. These institutes were economical in comparison to the hospitals and provided a service somewhere in between the workhouse and the Voluntary hospital. Doctors worked for free, which contributed to their prestige and may have increased their income from private patients. Dispensaries also provided a valuable training experience for doctors, who often dealt with people whose illnesses would not be allowed into the voluntary hospitals – such as infectious cases, or hopeless cases where patients were too ill to leave their homes. In housebound cases, dispensary doctors would visit to diagnose and treat the patient, but only if they lived within 'the dispensary area' and could produce a note from a subscriber. If they could not, then they would be passed over to the care of the poor law – which generally meant admission to a workhouse. The NHS removed the need for the dispensaries, however volunteers do still play a role in modern health care today, with over 3 million people volunteering in acute trusts, taking on roles such as befriending, hospitality, entertainment and administrative support.

General Practice

Prior to the twentieth century, general practitioners worked privately, treating people who had the means to pay, often in their own homes. In 1911, the Chancellor of the Exchequer, Lloyd George, introduced the National Insurance Act, which was influential in the development of primary care. It aimed to relieve hardship among the working classes during periods of illness, and made health insurance compulsory for workers, contracting GPs to provide medical services for working people – but not for their families, who were still required to pay.

The Act meant that unemployed workers no longer had to turn to the stigmatised welfare provisions of the Poor Law. All workers who earned less than £160 a year paid 4 pence into the scheme, their employer paid 3 pence and general taxation paid 2 pence – 'ninepence for fourpence'. Workers were then entitled to take sick leave at 10 shillings a week for the first 13 weeks and 5 shillings a week for the next 13. They were given access to free treatment for tuberculosis, and treatment from a panel doctor (or GP) of their choosing when sick.

A sizeable portion of society were still required to pay for medical treatment, and hospital inpatient care was still not provided to insured workers, meaning that many people continued to experience considerable hardship, until the NHS was established.

My NHS Story

Dr Rose Singleton is a GP working in rural Cumbria, who reflects on her experiences of being a new GP in the NHS:

'In 1924, Dr. Andrew Manson, protagonist of AJ Cronin's novel *The Citadel**, arrived in South Wales to start the first job of his medical career as an assistant to a local GP, Dr Page. He was 24 years old, fresh from medical school in Edinburgh and eager to get started. His growing unease is described in the initial paragraphs, as it becomes clear that Dr Page is incapacitated by a 'far from recent' stroke, and since the departure of the previous assistant, his clinics have been run by his dispenser. As a new doctor, Andrew is thrust into taking on responsibilities far beyond his comfort zone and without a safety net if things go wrong. Although Andrew Manson is a fictional character, Cronin was a doctor qualifying in 1919, and the novel draws on some of his experiences working in a South Wales mining town in the early twentieth century.

'I qualified 90 years after Cronin and was a junior doctor for seven years before achieving my CCT (certificate of completion of training), allowing me to work independently as a General Practitioner. Post-graduate training of doctors within the NHS is now much better organised, and General Practice is recognised as a specialty in its own right. What happened to Andrew Manson simply wouldn't happen now, with doctors – and of course their patients – being much better off for it.

'Despite this passing of time and the vast improvements in training since 1924, some things don't change; Andrew describes the first

---

* The Citadel by AJ Cronin was ground-breaking when published in 1937 dealing with medical ethics and extolling the virtues of socialized medicine. It has been credited with laying the foundations for the formation of the NHS.

patient he sees in his new role, "conscious of his nervousness, his inexperience, his complete unpreparedness for such a task". Away from the bustling wards he felt isolated and under-confident and suddenly had the pressure of making a diagnosis and devising a treatment plan alone. There can't be a doctor who hasn't felt this way, and with each step up in role, from foundation doctor to Registrar, to GP or Consultant, the pressure intensifies and the same uncomfortable feelings come flooding back. The hardest jump to make for me was from GP Registrar to fully qualified GP. After seven years of having my work scrutinised, assessed, and ultimately supervised, I fledged as a GP in the autumn of 2016, tumbling from the safety of my training programme, headlong into independence, and without anyone watching my back. I was reading "H is for Hawk" by Helen Macdonald around that time and I found some unexpected parallels with my experience of starting out in "real" general practice. Her description of becoming an expert, albeit in the art of falconry, really helped me understand why it was so hard: "Being a novice is safe. When you are learning how to do something, you do not have to worry about whether or not you are good at it. But when you have done something, have learned how to do it, you are not safe anymore. Being an expert opens you up to judgement." Although I was always responsible for the decisions I made as a junior doctor, everything I did was under the umbrella of a supervising GP or Consultant and losing that cover upon gaining my CCT was acutely exposing. Any bad decisions, oversights, or mistakes I made from that point forwards would be judged in the context of an expert, a GP, and I could no longer rely on the safety of the novice.

'I remember my first patient as a new GP, it was a toddler with fever. Having worked in paediatrics and through training in general practice, this was a familiar presentation, but by acquiring the title of GP and without the comfort blanket of my trainer to bail me out if I lost confidence, it felt like I was right back at the start, exactly like Andrew Manson. I now also had a permanent job for the first time in my career, I wouldn't just move on after six months, my name appears on hospital letters and patient records and I am cherished by some patients as *their* GP. It was likely I would see the little girl and her family again (and indeed I have done), and I couldn't hide behind a cloak of anonymity, previously granted by rotational junior doctor jobs.

'Being a GP in a small town, and furthermore within the community where I live, has opened my eyes to a network of connections that link people and experiences inextricably to their illness and their wellness. I understand why a lady with terrible osteoarthritis won't accept a hip replacement when I meet her confused old dad, who can't manage without her. The teenager with panic attacks doesn't have to tell me she's worried about cancer, because I know that her school friend recently died from it. I'm starting to see things differently, to see beyond symptoms and diseases, to glimpse the human condition in a way I haven't understood it before. I'm not a medical student anymore, I don't need a proforma for history taking, I'm not a GP trainee, having to follow a defined pattern for communicating with patients, I've developed a relationship with my community, which allows me to understand them in ways that I could barely touch upon as trainee. The breadth of knowledge, understanding and experience is an incredible revelation, but of course it can also be devastating. Imagine a middle-aged lady who comes for advice, wondering why she is struggling to count out the change in her shop. I can smell cigarettes on her breath and notice her clubbed fingers. I can guess without needing tests that she probably has lung cancer with brain metastases. I can see the future; the terrible conversation with her and her family when I tell them the result of the chest x-ray, her agonising realisation that it can't be treated, her death. As her GP, I'll be there through all of it; liaising with her specialists, arranging her palliative care, writing her death certificate and comforting her family when it's all over.

'I continue to find general practice challenging, but incredibly rewarding. There are few jobs, even within medicine, where you can potentially make someone feel better every ten minutes. A good GP can't be replaced by a robot or an app and whilst easy access to good medical advice is important, the role of a GP is so much more than technical nous, the value of which was superbly described by the great medical educationalist William Osler, 'It is much more important to know what sort of a patient has a disease than what sort of a disease a patient has.' The future of the NHS will include gene therapy, robotic surgery and digital health, but someone still has to be there when technology can't be, and I hope that GPs will continue to provide the holistic cornerstone that the NHS so vitally needs, now, and for generations to come.'

Chapter 2

The Formation of the NHS

The NHS was born on 5 July 1948. Doctors, nurses, dentists, opticians, pharmacists and hospitals came together for the first time as one colossal UK organization, and the unveiling of a hugely ambitious plan to provide free healthcare for all. Aneurin 'Nye' Bevan, the health secretary recognised as its creator, formally launched the service at Trafford General Hospital (known at the time as Park Hospital) in Manchester. The first NHS patient to be treated was 13-year old Sylvia

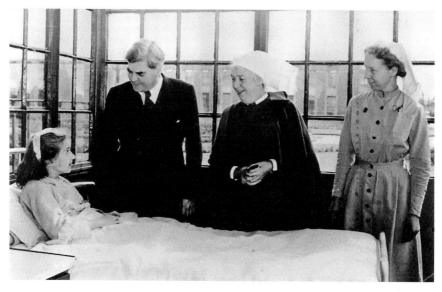

Aneurin Bevan, Minister of Health, on the first day of the National Health Service, 5 July 1948, at Park Hospital, Davyhulme, near Manchester. (via Wikimedia Commons)

Diggory, who recalls shaking Bevan's hand, saying, 'Mr Bevan asked me if I understood the significance of the occasion and told me that it was a milestone in history – the most civilised step any country had ever taken, and a day I would remember for the rest of my life – and of course, he was right.'

Aneurin Bevan

Aneurin Bevan, or Nye, as he was known, was born in a South Wales mining community in 1897. Growing up, he was exposed to poverty and disease, and three of his nine siblings died during childhood. His father was a coal miner, and Bevan followed in his footsteps, leaving school at age thirteen to work in the local colliery. His involvement in politics started as a miner, when he emerged as one of the leaders in the 1926 Miners' strike, and he was subsequently elected as a Labour MP. Bevan became well known as a champion for the working class, and he made an impression in parliament with his passionate debating style. Following Labour's landslide victory in 1945, he was appointed minister for health by Clement Atlee, and given the task of implementing the manifesto plans for a welfare state and healthcare revolution. Bevan recognised that health was a key factor in social inequalities and made it his mission to tackle this head on.

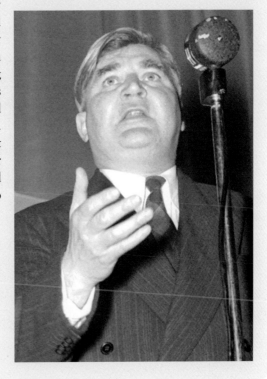

Aneurin Bevan.
(Geoff Charles via Wikimedia Commons)

Early twentieth century

The NHS was clearly not formed from thin air, but from an amalgamation of the healthcare services that already existed which, pre-1948, were messy and did not co-ordinate well together. The state had gradually taken responsibility for the health of the nation since the Poor Law reforms were implemented in Victorian Britain – leading to improved Public Health measures such as compulsory vaccination and surveillance of disease. Events such as the Boer War demonstrated that many people were unfit for active service. The dawn of the twentieth century welcomed a Liberal government who tried to reduce poverty and improve people's health by introducing reforms such as school medical inspections and free school meals. They introduced state funded pensions, initiated infant and maternal welfare clinics, and developed the health visitor system. Lloyd George's National Health Insurance scheme provided basic medical care to working men who paid their compulsory contributions to the scheme, providing the assurance of medical care should they

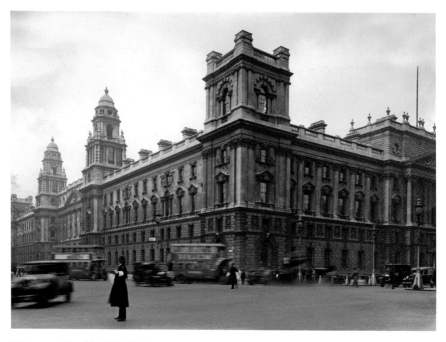

Ministry of health 1930. (Wellcome Collection)

become sick, and a limited income during periods of unemployment. Many resented giving up their hard-earned wages to such a scheme, and there remained glaring deficiencies to this system – such as a lack of access to hospital care, and an absence of universal cover for wives and children, who often continued to pay into private health insurance schemes.

The Ministry of Health was established in 1918, strengthening the philosophy that healthcare was the inherent responsibility of the state. The Ministry took control of the administration of the Poor Law, National Insurance, local government, planning, housing and environmental health. There were rumblings of discontent among the medical profession at the time of this slow expansion of state funded health services, and many saw it as a threat to their freedom to control their own incomes.

Lord Dawson's Report

In 1919, Sir Bertrand Dawson, a military doctor and physician at the London Hospital, was commissioned by the newly formed Ministry of Health to chair a council to advise on the systemized provision of health services to link the hospitals into a single system. His 1920 report outlined a model that would be adopted by the NHS 30 years later, based on primary healthcare centres, (staffed by general practitioners) and secondary health centres (hospitals staffed by consultant specialists). The committee's proposal was backed by a report eight years later from the Royal Commission on National Health Insurance who advocated for medical services to be divorced entirely from the insurance system in the same way as public health services – and funded by the general public's purse. The years following this saw a period of depression and economy cuts, which destroyed any chance of significant reform.

The state of healthcare

By the 1930s, many of the voluntary hospitals faced closure due to financial crises and many were pleading for state support. The charitable donations on which they depended reduced significantly over the years – in the 1890s, 88 per cent per cent of their income came from gifting, and this had dropped to a mere 35 per cent per cent by the 1930s, and many could not keep up with the costs of medical treatment. Furthermore, a national survey of hospitals was conducted in 1938 which indicated that the whole country needed an upgrade. The major problems identified were a shortage of beds due to poor hospital buildings, a shortage of consultants, and poor patient access to both. Lack of a structured system meant that the distribution of specialists around the country was haphazard. Complicated cases were cared for in hospitals without the necessary resources, and those hospitals that could deal with such cases had beds full of more simple cases. Long stay wards were lacking, some reported to have a ratio of 60 patients to 1 trained nurse, accommodating a mix of elderly patients with dementia on the same ward as young children. Furthermore, the cost of being sick was beyond the reach of the average person. A patient diagnosed with tuberculosis, undergoing operative treatment and several months bedrest would be expected to pay more than £1000.

The British Medical Association had proposed in 1930 that health insurance coverage should be given to the whole population, and that a co-ordinated regional hospital service should be instituted. The Socialist Medical Association went a step further and proposed that healthcare should be provided to all, free at the point of use, through a government led scheme. This policy for a state medical service was adopted by the Labour Party at their 1934 conference.

Wartime Healthcare

The threat of another war halted parliamentary discussions on the future of the health service and the Ministry turned their attention to co-ordinating all hospitals to join together to form an Emergency Medical Service (EMS) in preparation for the mass casualties of war. The number of beds in some hospitals was increased and temporary buildings were erected. Many of the former poor law institutions were upgraded, and many specialist centres (such as plastic surgery, neurosurgery and rehabilitation units) were created in preparation for war. The Ministry dictated what the functions of the existing hospital should be on a regional basis – which laid the foundation for a united health service when the war was over.

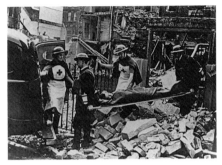 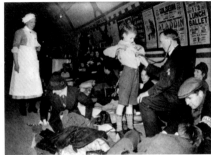

Above left: After an air raid. (Reproduced with permission from the British Red Cross Museum and Archives)

Above right: Piccadilly underground during the Blitz. (Reproduced with permission from the British Red Cross Museum and Archives)

Voluntary Aid Detachment

During the First World War, the British Red Cross set up the Voluntary Aid Detachment Scheme, and recruited thousands of women volunteers to serve their country providing nursing care. These civilian nurses sought employment in hospitals after the war, ultimately leading to the Registration of Nurses Act in 1919, which only allowed nurses with at least three years formal training to be admitted onto the nursing register.

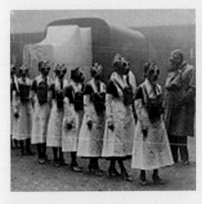 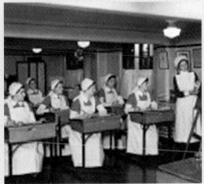

(Liverpool Nurses League)

The war changed attitudes. The state had controlled most aspects of people's lives during the war – with good effects. Rationing improved the health of the poor, and the EMS response to treating the casualties of air raids had given citizens access to healthcare that they had never experienced before – so the prospect of the government looking after healthcare did not seem outlandish. The major political parties largely agreed on the country's main priorities and generally cooperated to achieve them – namely post-war recovery and the welfare of the people – and the first twinklings of the NHS.

The Beveridge Report

The Beveridge report of 1942 set out plans for the future of post-war Britain and paved the way for the modern welfare state. Senior civil servant Sir William Beveridge chaired the committee tasked with reviewing social insurance schemes, and the resulting work 'Report on Social Insurance and Allied Services' became more succinctly known as the Beveridge Report. It put forward a scheme of ideas to tackle what he described as the 'five giant evils' that blighted the lives of British people: want; disease; ignorance; squalor and idleness. It advocated a compulsory social security scheme that would provide benefits without means testing. It proposed that all working people should pay a contribution to a state fund that could be used for a comprehensive health service, the avoidance of mass unemployment and a system of children's allowances. The report had piqued media curiosity and was published for public consumption, selling over 600,000 copies.

The white paper 'A National Health Service' was published in 1944 outlining the wartime coalition government's vision for a free, unified health service. It proposed central government management, with responsibility for its provision lying with the minister for health. The minister appointed to this position was Aneurin Bevan, whose proposals for the service went further than what had been discussed before, making him the almost single-handed architect of the NHS. In keeping with Labour's commitment to a programme of public ownership, he wanted nationalisation of municipal and voluntary hospitals with funding to come primarily from taxation rather than National Insurance. This regional hospital scheme to replace the local authority boundaries was a shrewd plan, as it meant the control of the hospitals would no longer be so insular, and executive control of all the hospitals would allow for service planning. In 1946, the National Health Service Act received Royal assent.

Structure of the new NHS

The NHS was planned as a three-tier service, with the Minister of Health overseeing it at the top, and three tiers which could interact with each other to suit the needs of the patient to include:

- Hospitals – Both the municipal and voluntary hospitals were nationalised and organised into 14 regional groups, or hospital boards.
- Primary Care – GPs, dentists, pharmacists and opticians all remained as self-employed professionals, contracted (by local executive councils) to provide services to the NHS so that the patient did not have to pay directly.
- Local Authority services – Community services (such as the provision of midwifery and health visiting services, school medical services, ambulance services, immunisation and public health) remained the responsibility of the local authorities.

Unhappy Doctors

Hospitals in 1948 were in a poor condition following war time bombing. Most had been built in the late 1800s and were beginning to crumble even before the Blitz. As previously mentioned, there was no sort of health system at the time and hospitals had been established over the years in a haphazard fashion. Most relied on GPs and unpaid consultants, who worked for free in exchange for a secure base for private practice.

The relationship between the medical profession and the state has always been guarded. Many doctors were opposed to the establishment of the NHS as they disliked the idea of becoming employees of the state, and the BMA led a vigorous campaign against it, some even comparing Bevan's proposals to Nazi Germany. Hospital doctors relied on private patients to boost their income and were wary of a new system that would endanger this. Bevan was famously reported as 'stuffing their mouths with gold' by allowing consultants to work within the NHS on a salaried basis (plus merit awards) but able to continue to do some lucrative private work within NHS hospitals. Proposals to make GPs salaried were declined and instead they reached a compromise in which they worked for the NHS as private contractors and were paid on a capitation basis, based on the number of patients they had on their list.

The Birth of the NHS

On 5 July 1948 medical care in the UK became free, for all people including foreigners living temporarily in Britain. Overnight, Bevan was in charge of 2688 hospitals in the UK, describing the new NHS as 'the most civilised step any country has ever taken'. In spite of the bickering, almost everyone was prepared to make the NHS work. 'The war made us realise that we were all neighbours'.

Additional resources for the new NHS were negligible. The same number of doctors and nurses went to work in the same hospitals on 5 July in the same way they had the day before, but what had changed was improved accessibility for patients and a more equitable distribution of existing services. *The Times* commented that the masses had joined the middle classes.

Demand for the NHS exceeded all predictions. During planning, the predicted annual cost was £170million. In its first full year of operation, costs exceeded £305 million. £1 million was budgeted for opticians, but within a year 5.25 million spectacle prescriptions had produced a bill amounting to £32 million. Similarly with prescriptions – in 1947, doctors issued 7 million prescriptions each month, which rose to 19 million per month by 1951.

Commentators in the BMJ in 1949 predicted the rate of NHS expenditure would lead to national ruin. They reasoned that the predicted NHS budgets planned for before its initiation had ignored the effects of the aging population and the figures were based on a false conception of health – meaning that before the NHS, people were cured of simpler and cheaper diseases but fell victim to more complex and more expensive diseases – for which the NHS was now footing the bill.

In 1950, Prime Minister Clement Atlee promoted Hugh Gaitskell to be Chancellor of the Exchequer. To balance the budget, he proposed savings of £13 million annually by imposing charges for dentures and spectacles provided by the NHS. Both Nye Bevan and Harold Wilson resigned from government the very next day in protest. The Conservative government went on to introduce charges for prescriptions of one shilling in 1952.

YOUR NEW
NATIONAL HEALTH SERVICE

On 5th July the new National Health Service starts

Anyone can use it—men, women and children. There are no age limits, and no fees to pay. You can use any part of it, or all of it, as you wish. Your right to use the National Health Service does not depend upon any weekly payments (the National Insurance contributions are mainly for cash benefits such as pensions, unemployment and sick pay).

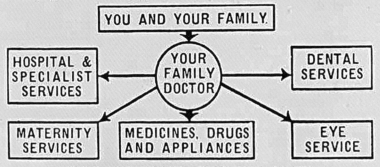

CHOOSE YOUR DOCTOR NOW

The first thing is to link up with a doctor. When you have done this, your doctor can put you in touch with all other parts of the Scheme as you need them. Your relations with him will be as now, *personal and confidential.* The big difference is that the doctor will not charge you fees. He will be paid, out of public funds to which all contribute as taxpayers.

So *choose your doctor now.* If one doctor cannot accept you, ask another, or ask to be put in touch with one by the new "Executive Council" which

has been set up in your area (you can get its address from the Post Office).

If you are already on a doctor's list under the old National Health Insurance Scheme, and do not want to change your doctor, you need *do nothing.* Your name will stay on his list under the new Scheme.

But make arrangements for *your family* now. Get an application form E.C.1 for *each* member of the family either from the doctor you choose, or from any Post Office, Executive Council Office, or Public Library; complete them and give them to the doctor.

There is a lot of work still to be done to get the Service ready. If *you* make *your* arrangements in good time, you will be helping both yourself and your doctor.

──────── *Issued by the Department of Health for Scotland* ────────   A

This advertisement appears in selected Sunday, Morning and Evening newspapers in Scotland.

National Health Service leaflet May 1948. (via Wikimedia commons)

Apart from a period between 1965 and 1968, prescription charges in England have continued ever since. Today, prescriptions cost £8.80 per item and provide an estimated £450 million revenue for the NHS annually. A system of exemptions* for prescription charges is in place, including those on low incomes, pensioners and students, pregnant women and people with long term medical conditions, meaning than on average 90 per cent per cent of all NHS prescriptions are dispensed free of charge. There are growing concerns about wastage of medications prescribed for free, which in 2009 was estimated in the region of £150million of avoidable waste.

General Practitioners

Before 1948, GPs worked as independent traders treating people who had the money to pay them, often from a consulting room in their own home. In 1911, GPs were contracted by local insurance committees administering Lloyd George's National Insurance Scheme, to provide general medical services, and were paid a capitation fee for every patient registered with them. At the inception of the NHS, this independent contractor status was clung to, from a fear of becoming a salaried employee of the state, but this independence was deceptive. GPs continued to be free to organise their own practices, but the work they did for the NHS was controlled by a tightly defined contract. They received a capitation fee for each patient registered with them, and their expenses were averaged and included in this payment-per-patient. No money could pass between patient and doctor (with few exceptions such as payment for a private medical certificate). The NHS Act of 1946 had planned for health centres to be a main feature of primary care. They envisaged clinics aimed at health promotion made up of GPs, dentists and local health authority clinics, funded by the public purse – but this programme was aborted before it even started. Prior to the NHS, a few GPs had made a handsome living by treating wealthy private patients, but the majority were poorly paid, so the NHS provided them with security.

Lord Beveridge had predicted that the initial jump in demand for GPs' services would eventually fall once people became accustomed

---

* You can find out more about who is eligible for prescription exemptions here: https://www.nhs.uk/NHSEngland/Healthcosts/Pages/Prescription-costs.aspx

to the system, but this never happened, and GPs were overwhelmed with demands from patients who had previously avoided seeking care for financial reasons. Within a month, 90 per cent per cent of the population had registered with a GP. Each GP was personally responsible for the care of their patients 24 hours a day, 7 days a week, 365 days a year, meaning single handed doctors could be on call around the clock with no respite. GPs were assigned as the gatekeepers for the NHS, transferring the decision to go for hospital treatment from the patient to the doctor. A patient's guide produced by the Ministry of Health in 1948 declared that the GP would 'arrange for the patient every kind of specialist care he is himself unable to give. Except in emergency, hospital and specialists would not normally accept a patient for advice or treatment unless he has been sent by his family doctor'. This suited hospital consultants, who felt protected from 'trivial' cases. The government enjoyed increased cost effectiveness, while the GPs enjoyed the continuing responsibility for 'their' patients. This changed the relationship between GPs and consultants, who had previously relied on GP referral as a source of private income. Now they had plenty of NHS patients to keep them busy, few consultants made a substantial income privately and no longer had financial reasons to be grateful to GPs. In the current day debates about NHS privatisation, this statement frequently pops up, that 'GP's are private providers!' NHS GPs may be run as private businesses, but they differ from private GP practices in that they do not compete for patients or for profit. They work to NHS contracts, follow NHS guidelines, and see NHS patients.

Optometry

Ophthalmic services did not quite fit into the NHS plan. In 1948, most opticians based their business on the provision of spectacles. Many also provided sight tests, but at this time, there was a proportion of the medical profession who opposed the right of ophthalmic opticians to conduct eye examinations. Once the NHS introduced free eye testing there simply was not enough ophthalmologists in the country to meet the demand and opticians gladly took on this role. This eventually led to the profession being recognised with legislation in 1958 to regulate optical professionals in a similar way to doctors and dentists.

After 1948, an influx of patients attended for their free sight testing – many people demanding free spectacles, even when their vision was

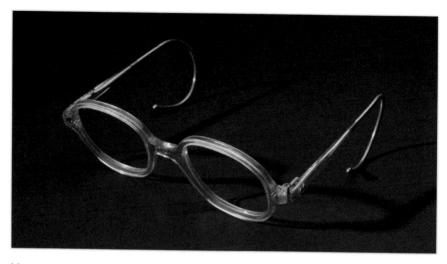

Mass produced spectacles were available in the UK in the 1950s and 1960s through the National Health Service. These frames are a typical example. The coil springs secured the frames when the arms hooked behind the ears. (Science Museum, London. Wellcome Images)

found to be perfect. By the end of the 1940s, waiting lists of 18 months for spectacles were commonplace, meaning by the time some received their devices, their vision had changed, and they had to return for an updated prescription. By 1950, this was costing the NHS £22 million annually, and in 1951, the end of free spectacles was one of the first cuts to be made in the NHS. The above image shows a typical pair of NHS glasses, which were almost universally loathed by the wearers due to the stigma attached to wearing state subsidised spectacles.

NHS spectacles showed little imagination in terms of design flair. They were made cheaply for robust use and utility rather than fashion.

History of Dentistry in the UK

Rewinding back a few hundred years, the introduction of sugar brought with it a rise in tooth decay and gum disease. Sugar was initially a luxury reserved only for the rich, some even brushed their teeth with honey and sugar paste, and indeed, Queen Elizabeth I was rumoured to have blackened teeth and foul breath. Consumption increased in the general population throughout the eighteenth century as people developed a taste for toffees, fudge and jams – creating a demand for dental care. During this period, they had several options for their toothache. They could turn to the local blacksmith, who was always happy to pull a tooth, they had the barbers and barber surgeons and they also had the travelling tooth drawers. The tooth drawers are considered to be the forefathers of modern dentistry, since they made a living solely from treating teeth. They travelled the country, attracting trade by putting on a show in the market square, dressing as jesters and wearing necklaces of teeth, then they would extract the teeth of willing participants for a fee in full view of the assembled villagers. The role of these 'operators of the teeth' grew to not only removing teeth, but making artificial teeth, and early methods used a carved hippopotamus ivory base, with human teeth riveted in. The source of the human teeth was dubious – they were notably taken from the mouths of dead soldiers from battlefields such as Waterloo, but as demand grew, they were acquired from dissecting rooms, mortuaries and even graveyards. Dentures were extremely expensive and reserved for the higher echelons of society. By the nineteenth century, dentistry had become a respected profession, and in attempts to distinguish medically trained dentists with quacks such as jewellers who often gave it a go as a lucrative side line, the Royal College of Surgeons instituted a qualification in dentistry, which led to regulation in the same way as doctors.

The importance of good oral hygiene gained attention at the start of the twentieth century. During recruitment for the British army for the Boer War, general poor health had been highlighted, but dental hygiene especially was noted to be dire. From a force of over 200,000 soldiers, there were nearly 7000 admissions to hospital due to dental causes. Strong teeth were essential to tear the rifle paper needed to load a musket, leading to the expression 'You can't fight if you can't bite!' During the First World War, soldiers were issued with toothbrushes – but had allegedly used them to clean their boots instead. The importance of dental care for the troops was recognised which eventually led to the formation of the Army Dental Corps in 1921. The facial trauma seen during the world wars led to the establishment of specialist oral surgery units. Access to dental care for civilians was lacking and most people avoided a visit until pain forced them into the dentist's chair. When plans were being formed for the NHS, the Friendly and Approved Societies set up under the 1911 National Insurance acts shared their figures, which showed that in the 1930s, only 27 per cent per cent of the UK population accessed regular dental care. The government were keen for this to improve, and launched health education campaigns, proclaiming in a 1944 report 'The British Public is ill educated and apathetic in regards to the care of the teeth. This attitude springs mainly from the national fear of pain and lack of any real understanding of the importance of dental health'. They were keen to change habits to encourage people to visit the dentist for regular inspections rather than when prompted by pain.

Water Fluoridisation

The use of fluoride proved one of the most effective public health improvements of the twentieth century in reducing tooth decay. Its discovery can be traced back to Colorado Springs, in 1908, when a local dentist noticed that people living in this area has less decay than those in the neighbouring villages. Analysis of the water supply showed high levels of fluoride. Artificial fluoridation of water supply was introduced in the states in 1945, and trialled in the UK, in Birmingham in 1964. Fluoride based toothpastes were launched in the early 1960's, and mass scale production followed in the 1970's.

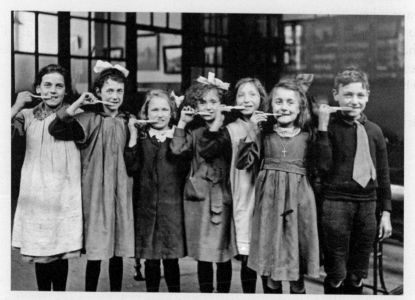

Toothbrush Drill at School – England circa 1920. (From the Wellcome Collection)

NHS Dentistry

When dental care was included in NHS provisions in 1948, demand for treatment was overwhelming. Reports spoke of dentists seeing over a hundred patients a day as people flocked in to sort out their previously neglected not so pearly whites. Surgeries were open seven days a week, and patients still had to be turned away. At the end of the first year, many dentists were earning £4000 a year after expenses (compared to roughly £1400 before 1948 – and almost double that of the average family doctor during the same period). Restrictions were later introduced to reduce pay-outs over a specified level.

Prior to free dental treatment, it was common to be given a set of dentures as a wedding present – patients would have all of their teeth extracted in favour of a complete set of fake choppers, which avoided multiple future trips to the dentist. In the first nine months of the NHS, 33 million sets of artificial teeth had been provided by NHS dentists. Everyone wanted a pair. Not just one pair – often two, or three sets since they weren't paying for them. This figure had reached 66 million between 1950 and 1951, putting such a drain on the NHS, that the first charges were introduced.

Charges have increased since then, and various service re-organisations have taken place, resulting in an NHS service in which patients have to contribute towards the cost of care. Some dentists remarked that they had never been a part of the NHS in the same way as GPs, who received capitation payments for all patients registered on their lists, while dentists were contractors who were paid on a fee for service basis.

As of April 2016, there were three standard charges for all NHS dental treatments in England and Wales:

- Band 1 course of treatment – £20.60 in England, £13.50 in Wales; covers an examination, diagnosis (including X-rays), advice on how to prevent future problems, a scale and polish if needed, and application of fluoride varnish or fissure sealant. Band 1 also covers emergency care needed for trauma and severe pain or swelling, even if more than one visit is required.
- Band 2 course of treatment – £56.30 in England (Wales: £43.00) covers everything listed in Band 1, plus fillings, root canal work or removal of teeth.

- Band 3 course of treatment – £244.30 (Wales: £185.00) covers everything listed in Bands 1 and 2, plus crowns, dentures and bridges.

Dentists are paid in 'Units of Dental Activity', typical values being £20-35. They are paid one UDA for a band 1 course of treatment, three for a band 2, and twelve for a band 3 course of treatment. Patient charges are deducted from these values meaning that for many treatments, the rate of pay is below the cost of actually providing the treatment and as a result, many dentists will refer patients elsewhere for treatments that will not provide them with a profit.

In 2016, the British Dental Association (BDA) released figures showing that dental charges had pushed 600,000 patients with dental problems to see already overstretched GPs, unequipped to provide dental treatment, costing £26 million in wasted GP appointments. One in five patients had reportedly postponed dental treatment due to concerns about costs and based on the current trajectory of dental charge increases, it is estimated that by the year 2032, patient charges will actually exceed the funding provided by the government in the NHS dental budget.

It is a sad fact that the NHS has betrayed its founding principles and is simply not free at the point of use for dental care, resulting in a service that is isolating many patients. Charities such as Dentaid now operate in some parts of the UK to provide free care where dental waiting lists are long and people are unable to access NHS dentists. The state of NHS finances means that the rest of healthcare is in danger of suffering the same fate.

My NHS Story

Kate Cavanagh is a UK Veterinary Surgeon and reflects on her experiences of customers paying for care for their pets

'Most veterinary care throughout the developed world is given through private practices owned by individuals or partners. Prices vary due to area, experience of staff, amenities and reputation but are largely in the control of the owner(s). In recent years corporate chains have surfaced, buying out many of the independent practices and bringing a more standardised pricing system. I qualified as a Veterinary Surgeon 15 years ago. For many years I worked as an assistant at various private practices in the UK around the Northwest and Midlands.

'You may wonder what this has to do with the NHS. Eight years ago, I moved to a niche area of our profession – the charity sector. I would like to share with you some of my personal reasons for this switch, and how I see similarities between the veterinary sector and medical sector. Perhaps lessons can be learnt from the smaller-scale veterinary profession.

'I work for a charity aiming to serve those on the bottom financial rung of UK society. We encourage donations for treatment, but it is effectively free treatment at the point of service, similar to the NHS. To our clients, our service is often seen as a sort of NHS for their pets. However, we are entirely charity financed, mainly through the giving of legacies and have no government funding. I guess you could say, like the NHS, we are spending other people's money, so are duty bound to make best use of it.

'Throughout my career in private practice I was exposed to what I can only describe as the monetisation of life and death. Pet insurance is not mandatory. Owners who do not have insurance (or have insurance that does not cover that situation or have it perhaps where the limit has been reached), are faced with the daunting prospect that they may not be able to afford treatment for their pet. Consultations can be a relentless battle between what we should do and what we can do. Discussions regarding costs can take the limelight instead of the animal. The challenge of trying to maintain clinical standards and integrity whilst staying within each owner's budget was often the hardest aspect of the job. It could end in following a treatment route that is far from ideal, or ultimately, premature euthanasia of the pet on financial grounds.

'A case I remember well was that of a young Yorkshire Terrier named Betty. She was forever trying to make friends with the neighbour's cat. The feeling was not mutual, and after the most recent altercation, a scratch on her eye developed into an ulcer. It did not respond well to treatment and in the end the only option was to remove the eye. Even at a very heavily discounted price (zero profit) the owner could still not finance it, and at a later date she was euthanised. An awful situation for that pet owner and the vet involved, knowing that something could be done but finances prevented it. Not charging appropriately may ease the conscience but the business would not last long.

'Situations like that of Betty can cause feelings of guilt and anger. I have heard colleagues being called murderers and face verbal and physical abuse. Occasionally we personally take on the animals and associated costs using our own money. Many vets end up with a 'rescue', which are often three-legged, or one-eyed, or missing something! Sadly, this cannot be the case every time. The toll on vets, who are often deeply compassionate and caring people, and the ones holding that last needle, is often forgotten.

'The daily struggle with situations like this was part of why I left private practice to work in the charity sector. As a doey eyed, animal loving, James Herriot addicted, 12 year old, I had not thought about this side of the job. Of course, in my current job we have to make sensible decisions with our funds, I suppose in the same way the NHS does. But clinical standards are good and Betty's situation would never happen. We treat dozens of animals just like her every day. I wonder in the USA and other countries, where there is a limited social medical care system, how many difficult decisions patients, relatives and doctors have to make due to finances. Thanks to the NHS it is an added angle that we don't have to worry about. The prospect of that changing scares me. It is traumatic having these discussions over a much loved pet but imagine if a similar scenario played out at your next appointment in the GP or with a doctor about a sick relative. Unimaginable.

'The subject of veterinary bills comes up a lot, many telling me how astounded they are at bills they receive for veterinary care. I wonder if many consider the cost of their own healthcare. If so, would they find vets' bills so shocking? Prices do vary nationally, but at my local private veterinary practice a consultation with medication costs around £50-60. I don't know what the equivalent GP consult with medicine costs. Perhaps we should all know the answer to this.* Vets often use similar equipment and medicines, often sending samples to the same laboratories for testing. I remember, during my university days before MRI scanners were commonplace in veterinary medicine, lurking behind the human MRI scanner on Crown Street in Liverpool waiting for the humans to leave before we could use the scanner for our furry patients.

---

* According to the Personal Social Services Research Unit (PSSRU) the cost of an 11.7 minute face to face GP consultation (excluding direct care staff costs and without qualification costs) in 2015 was £33. http://www.pssru.ac.uk/project-pages/unit-costs/2017

Do people know how much an MRI scan costs? An X-ray? A course of physiotherapy? I hear complaints about prescription charges. If the real cost of the medicine people are taking were known, perhaps they would consider it a steal. Expectations and longevity have increased, with more people wanting 'Supervet' style treatment without the price tag. Perhaps this is true of my counterparts in the medical profession.

'We price up the work we perform, as we would for a paying client, and present this itemised "dummy" bill to the client. It gives them an idea of how much the care of their pet would have cost, were they not eligible to use our service. The aim being to raise awareness of veterinary costs and also encourage donations. Perhaps doing this for healthcare would help raise awareness of how much our healthcare really costs. It would also help people see that veterinary charges are fair.

'I feel hugely grateful to have a National Health Service, and to those that work to keep it grinding on day by day. Perhaps I have seen in some small way some of the effects privatisation would have for patients and workers. I will continue to both celebrate it and protect it with pride wherever I can. Although we already have many fabulous human medical charities to cover gaps in funding, I suppose without a National Health Service style system, charities like my own would be needed to rescue those on that bottom financial rung of society.'

A Different World: 1948 vs 2018

When the NHS began in 1948, the UK population stood at 49.4 million. 70 years later in 2018, the population is estimated at 66.5 million. By 2068 this is predicted to grow to 82 million. There are an estimated 3million people with diabetes in England, and 26 per cent per cent of both men and women are now classified as obese. The population is expected to continue to age with the number of people over 60 expected to rise from 14.9m in 2014 to 21.9m by 2039 – all which will have implications for healthcare.

- Life expectancy – In 1948 the life expectancy for men was 66 and for women, 71. Today, men can expect to live to the age of 79.2 and women 82.9
- Infant mortality – In 1948 there were 34.5 deaths per 1000 live births. Today that figure is 3.7

- Death – In 1948, the main killers were rheumatic heart disease (almost unheard of today) circulatory disorders and infection. Over the past 70 years, the proportion of deaths caused by cancer has risen (in line with an aging population), while those caused by tuberculosis and respiratory disease have fallen.
- In 1948, 65 per cent per cent of Britain's population smoked. Figures from 2013 show that this number has dropped to less than 20 per cent per cent
- In 1948, the annual cost of the NHS per head, per lifetime was £200. Today that figure has risen to £2106
- The NHS was launched with 68,013 hospital staff (excluding doctors). In March 2017, the NHS employed 106,430 doctors, 285,893 nurses, 21,597 midwives, 132,673 technical staff, 19,772 ambulance staff, 21,139 managers and 9974 senior managers
- In 1950, there were approximately 21,450 GPs in Britain. In March 2017 there were 33,423 full time GPs (excluding locums) – a reduction of 890 from 2016
- Today, the NHS sees 1 million patients every 36 hours

Chapter 3

Timeline of the NHS

1950s

The first decade of the NHS was not without its problems, but it was successful enough to cement it into an institution. A free, universal service was a huge cultural change from what had preceded it, and only three years into the NHS, financial challenges became evident resulting in the introduction of charges for prescriptions, dental and optical services by the end of 1952. The fifties saw a post war baby boom and the introduction of technologies such as the microwave oven, plastics, nylon stockings and computers. Medical technological also thrived. Ultrasound was adapted for use in foetal monitoring and the success of antibiotics in the 1940s was followed by a rash of new drugs. Cortisone was discovered in 1950 as were the thiazides for hypertension and the first effective remedies for tuberculosis were introduced. Antipsychotics such as chlorpromazine and haloperidol were synthesized, the use of blood products became more common and interferon was discovered. The Thalidomide tragedy started in 1958, when pregnant women were prescribed the medication as a tranquilliser – only to find in the 1960s that it was responsible for causing severe birth defects. In 1954, in the USA, the food preservative BHA (butylated hydroxyanisole) was approved (the same year that McDonalds was franchised) signalling the growth of fast food chains, ready-made meals and the start of the obesity epidemic.

1950   **The link between smoking and lung cancer is proven.** Richard Doll had been studying lung cancer patients since the 1940s, expecting to find it was caused by fumes from coal fires or cars, but instead found that smokers are more likely to die of lung cancer than non-smokers. He also found an increased risk of heart disease. Doll quit smoking during his study and lived to the age of 92.

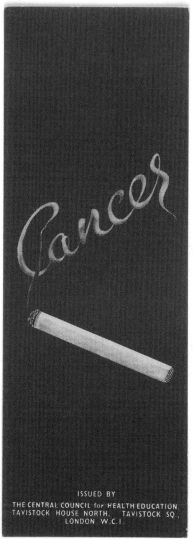

The Dangers of smoking. (Taken from the Wellcome Collection)

The Collings Report – the first major report on quality in general practice – found poor standards of care, poor working conditions and isolation from other professionals. GPs had remained outside of the NHS as independent contractors rather than salaried employees. The 1948 NHS Act had intended that GPs would move away from being single handed, and would be rehoused with other GPs inside health centres, but this proved unaffordable.

Labour government

1951   **Charges for dental and optical appliances imposed**
        Conservative government

1952   **Prescription charges** of one shilling are introduced and a flat rate of £1 for ordinary dental treatment
        College of General Practitioners formed
        Watson and Crick discover structure of the DNA (Deoxyribonucleic acid). DNA makes up our genes, which pass on hereditary characteristics from parent to child. Knowing the structure of this set the foundations for the study of genetic diseases.

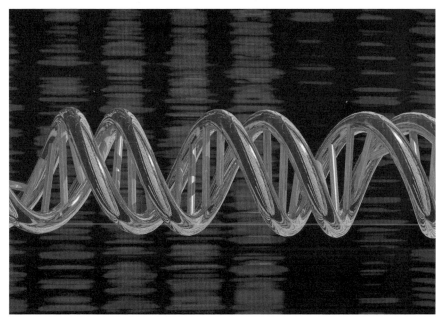

DNA double helix and sequencing output. (Peter Artymiuk, Wellcome Collection)

1953 Coronation of Queen Elizabeth II
Summit of Everest climbed for the first time by Sir Edmund Hillary and Tenzing Norgay

1954 **Children are granted daily visits** from their families while in hospital. Until this time, visiting was only permitted for an hour at the weekend. Children were often placed alone in adult wards, with little explanation as to what was happening to them. Paediatricians realised that this separation was traumatic and instituted family visiting.
Rationing ends
The Percy Commission is established by Winston Churchill's government to review the care given to people with mental health problems. They recommend that treatment should be given in the community where possible, rather than in large

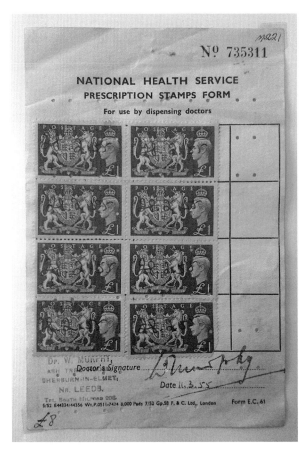

NHS Prescription Stamps. (via Wikimedia Commons)

psychiatric institutions. This is supported by the 1959 Mental Health Act, which also states that mentally ill patients should not be differentiated from physically sick patients.

1956 **The Guillebaud Report** on the cost of the NHS is published. It reports that the cost of the NHS in relative terms is falling and that capital spending is 33 per cent per cent of pre-war levels and that future costs would be met by economic growth.

The Clean Air Act is passed, aimed at reducing the air pollution created by burning coal. In 1952, a 'Great Smog' descended upon London, exacerbating the health problems of those with heart and lung conditions, resulting in a dramatic increase in mortality rates. The act allowed local authorities to control emissions from industrial premises and improved death rates

1957 **The Willick Report** suggests a 12 per cent per cent reduction in the number of doctors being trained, due to the increasing numbers of specialist registrars unable to secure specialist

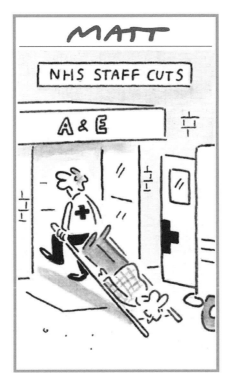

(© Telegraph Media Group Limited)

consultant posts. This is later considered a misjudgement, and training numbers are increased in 1961. The report is retrospectively believed to be responsibility for the severe shortages of junior medical staff throughout the 1960s.

1958   **Polio and Diptheria vaccination programme launched** ensuring everyone under 15 is vaccinated, leading to a dramatic reduction in cases

The Opticians Act allows opticians to become regulated professionals

My NHS Story

Meg Parkes is an Honorary Research Fellow at the Liverpool School of Tropical Medicine. She trained as a nurse in the 1970s and reflects on her NHS experiences

'I was born into the NHS in 1953: I was 0, it was nearly 5. I grew up in it, the daughter of two General Practitioners who worked tirelessly for the benefit of others. It helped to shape me. After leaving school, I first trained as a medical secretary and then applied to train as a general nurse. During the secretarial course I gained a broader understanding of the local NHS services – GPs' surgeries, local clinics and administration.

'I began three years of adult State Registered Nurse (SRN) training in September 1972 at Manchester Royal Infirmary (MRI). It was an apprenticeship and we had to live-in for the first year of training; all uniform was provided – cotton dresses, cuffs, collars, caps and capes and of course, starched aprons – and laundered by the hospital. Nurses' Homes were run by wardens and we had single rooms off long, deep carpeted corridors (to ensure quiet for those on night duty) at the end of which were the bathrooms, each with cast iron baths the size of small troop carriers. The hot water was never ending... what bliss!

'Pre-NHS MRI had been a voluntary hospital (funded by public subscription), the city's premier university teaching hospital. An air of excellence pervaded the wards and its endless miles of corridors; those of us accepted for training were encouraged to feel part of an elite and were expected to maintain the reputation and dignity of the hospital. I certainly felt very privileged to be there. After an eight-week introductory course we nurse chicks were let loose on unsuspecting wards full of patients. This was where our apprenticeships really began, learning from the senior students and qualified staff by observing, before eventually being allowed to try. In between times we took temperatures and cleaned anything that stood still. Our 12-week placements included time in medicine, surgery, orthopaedics and gynaecology – each followed by two-week blocks, known as School, where we had lectures and practical training.

'My first month's salary, with tax, NI and living-in charges deducted, was £48. For this I had worked five eight-hour day shifts per week. Early shifts started at 7.30am, lates at 12.30pm, with the dreaded split shifts – in at 7.30, off at 1pm, back in at 4pm till 9pm – whenever the rota dictated. After just six months' training we were eligible for the night rota: 11-hour shifts from 9pm – 8am worked over a fortnight. It was common to work 10 nights on followed by four off. Though responsibility on nights was enormous we survived, as did most of our patients.

'On qualifying and promotion to Staff Nurse, we were expected to work at the hospital for at least a further year to earn our Hospital Badge (at MRI this was a large, distinctive and much-coveted bronze penny). Regrettably it was not for me. Due to ill-health, I had to defer my training for 18 months and spent time working as the manager of a General Practice, seeing the NHS from a different perspective.

'I eventually completed my training at what were then known as Hope Hospital and Salford Royal, and came to realise this change of hospitals helped broaden my outlook. Hope Hospital was, pre-NHS, a municipal hospital (former Poor Law, or Work House hospital). It was more "local" than MRI in every sense – patients, staff, nursing experience. While serious or unusual cases were routinely referred to MRI, there was still plenty of acute medicine and surgery to keep us busy.

'One stark memory of my student days was that we were always rushed off our feet. We never felt we had enough time to give our patients the care we knew they needed. Wards were often short staffed, especially during winters and compromise was the order of the day: 'prioritise the urgent and do the best you can for the rest' was a constant mantra. We felt really embattled at times. Sound familiar?

'Another lasting memory was when, towards the end of my first year, I got engaged. I was summoned before MRI's formidable Matron, a highly-acclaimed nurse with a fearsome reputation. She quizzed me about my determination to complete my training, told me that the hospital's needs were my priority and whether I got the day off to get married was entirely in the hands of the sister in charge of the ward! I did, but only because I had temporarily left training. I knew one student who worked a split shift on her wedding day.

'After qualifying I returned briefly, as a Staff Nurse on nights at a local general hospital. I vividly remember on one shift a boorish patient berating me for being late to answer a patient's bell. Myself and the auxiliary were busy at the other end of the ward and I had responded as soon as I could. He loudly demanded better service for himself and his fellow patients, ending his rant by stating dramatically, "I pay my stamp. I am entitled to a proper service, it's my right!" I looked him in the eye and said calmly, "Your stamp won't buy the floor tile you're standing on." As I walked across to the patient who had really needed my attention applause broke out around me.

'I look back on my all too brief years of nursing with gratitude for such a valuable training for life. What a privilege it is to care for others when they are most in need. Having four children put paid to my return to nursing, shifts even in the late 1980s were not family friendly.

'Now in my mid-60s, I believe my generation has been the most fortunate in every sense: born into a country that was free, with free education, healthcare, almost unlimited choices and the chance of a decent pension. We should remember that. Stop moaning about 'the broken NHS', give thanks and do something useful, like paying for services when we can afford to, so it can work better. What finer legacy could we leave our families.'

1960s

The buoyant economy of the technicolour sixties brought low unemployment rates and increasing affluence. UK families bought their first cars, kitchen appliances and televisions, and mass communication became a reality. Music and fashion defined the era, and rebellious lyrics against the authorities fostered young people to stand up for their beliefs and individuality. Sixties teenagers were the first generation free from conscription and the decade saw laws regarding divorce, homosexuality and abortion become more liberalized. Feminism gained credibility meaning women could broaden their dreams beyond motherhood and marriage. In 1968, 850 female factory workers in Dagenham went on strike, fighting for equal pay to their male co-workers – and the Equal Pay Act was passed in 1970 as a result. The newly introduced contraceptive pill created a sexual revolution, while a boom in pharmaceuticals saw the development of drugs of abuse: Valium to soothe the nerves of housewives and psychotropic drugs such as LSD which helped bring about the 'hippie' movement. Immigration brought with it foreign imports such as spaghetti Bolognese and chicken tikka masala, forever changing the nation's eating habits. Immigration also bolstered the workforce of the NHS. The Caribbean and Ireland had been a primary source of nurses since the 1940s, in the 1960s more than 18,000 doctors came from Indian and Pakistan in response to an appeal by health minister Enoch Powell. NHS inefficiencies were apparent in the sixties and a system of health authorities was proposed to replace the disjointed tripartite system; this eventually came into being in the seventies.

1960   **Male nurses** are admitted to the Royal College of Nursing for the first time. When registration for nurses was introduced in 1919, trained male nurses (who often worked in asylums) were not able to join and were kept on a supplementary register until 1960.

Surgical Firsts. The first UK kidney transplant is performed by Michael Woodruff in Edinburgh. The 49-year-old twins both survive for six years, before dying of an unrelated illness. In the same year, the first full hip replacement is carried out at the Wrightington Hospital by Professor John Charnley. He asks

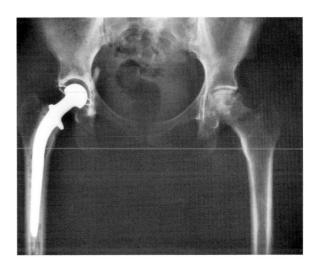

Pelvic xray showing
a total hip joint
replacement, (via
Wikimedia Commons)

patients if they mind returning their hips to him post mortem, and the majority agree, allowing him to check for wear and tear and research improved future models.

1961   **The oral contraceptive pill is launched,** and is hailed as a twentieth century breakthrough, playing a role in liberating women and enabling greater sexual freedom. For the first time, sex was effectively separated from reproduction, allowing childbirth to be planned around careers, resulting in a reduction in early marriages, and increase in female university enrolment. It has prompted both health scares and moral debates since its introduction. Initially it is only offered to married women, but this is relaxed in 1967, and by 1969, almost 1 million women are using it. Provision of contraception was initially the work of charitable organisations such as the Family Planning Association and Marie Stopes, but once it became available on NHS prescription, patients increasingly obtained it from their GP. All forms of contraception remain free in the UK today on the NHS. Patients in the USA can pay up to $50 per month for birth control pills and up to $1300 to have an intrauterine contraceptive device (IUD) inserted.

Enoch Powell's Water Tower Speech is seen as a milestone in mental health service provision, speaking of an end to the old asylums and a move to greater community care

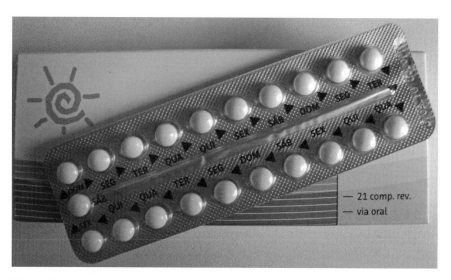

The oral contraceptive pill. (Beria L Rodriguez via Wikipedia Commons)

1962   The **Hospital Plan** approved the development of District General Hospitals for populations of around 125,000, in an attempt to unify the tripartite system of hospitals, GPs and local authorities, and make hospitals accessible to the populations they served. A ten year construction plan is put in place. New hospitals had not been built for many years prior to this and the costs and time involved in the redevelopment were grossly underestimated at the outset.

The Porritt Review is published the same year, led by old-school surgeon Sir Arthur Porritt. He was initially sceptical about the formation of NHS (and had been a critic in the 1940s), but had been convinced that it had to continue. He suggested the system was fragmented, and that Area Health Boards should be established to bring together hospital, GP and community services.

1964   **Water Fluoridation** is introduced to the water supply with the intention to reduce tooth decay
Labour government

1965   **Prescription Charges abolished**
Abolition of the Death Penalty
The Seebohm Committee is established and publish their report in 1968 reviewing the organization and responsibilities of the social services functions of the local authorities. They advise an amalgamation of welfare services, home help, mental health and social work services to create a unified department, able to support care in the community.

1966   A new contract **improved pay and conditions for GPs**, instituting a maximum list size of 2,000 patients, improving resources available for professional education and improvement in premises and hiring support staff. Following this, group practices became the norm.

1967   **The Salmon Report** makes recommendations for developing the nursing staff structure and the status of the profession in hospital management.
The Cogwheel Report considers the organization of doctors within hospitals and proposes speciality groupings
The Abortion Act is introduced by the Liberal MP David Steel and becomes law in 1968, allowing termination of pregnancy

by a registered physician up to 28 weeks gestation, if two other doctors agree that it is in the best mental and physical interests of the woman. In 1990, this is reduced to 24 weeks. In 2018, the Act still does not extend to Northern Ireland.

1968   **Britain's first heart transplant** is carried out in May 1968 by South African born surgeon Donald Ross in London. A team of eighteen spend seven hours on the procedure, on what is the tenth procedure of its kind carried out since the operation was pioneered by Christiaan Barnard in Cape Town, a year earlier. The patient dies after 46 days from an associated infection
Sextuplets born. After undergoing fertility treatment, a British woman gives birth to four girls and two boys at Birmingham maternity hospital, assisted by a team of twenty-eight. One of the girls dies at the birth and two more die later
Prescription charges reintroduced
The first green paper on the NHS is published, recommending the creation of 50 area boards in attempt to remedy the organizational deficiencies of the NHS. Governmental Green papers are typically consultation papers containing proposals for change, while White Papers are issued as statements of

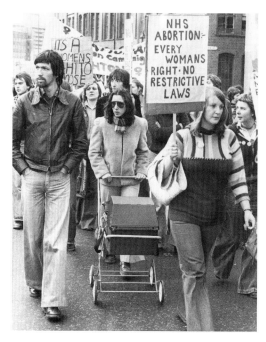

Pro-abortion protestors. (©Marx Memorial Library/Mary Evans)

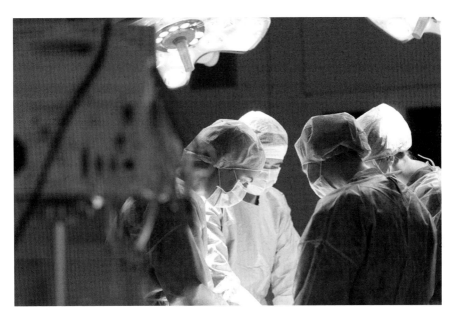

Group of surgeons in the operating room. (Adobe Stock Images)

policy and often set out changes for new legislation – known as a Bill, which is then debated in Parliament. When a Bill is given Royal Assent by the Queen, it becomes an Act – and thus Law **The Department of Health and Social Security** is formed from the merging of the Ministry of Health and the Ministry of Social Security

1969 **Man on the moon** – Buzz Aldrin and Neil Armstrong become the first men to step on the moon

The Liverpool School of Tropical Medicine and Far East Prisoners of War

The Liverpool School of Tropical Medicine (LSTM) had a long post-war collaboration with British ex-Far East Prisoners of War (FEPOWs). These men suffered from the consequences of captivity for decades after their release, many of them still experiencing relapses of amoebic dysentery and malaria many years later. From 1967 until 1999, LSTM was asked by the Department of Health to become the primary centre

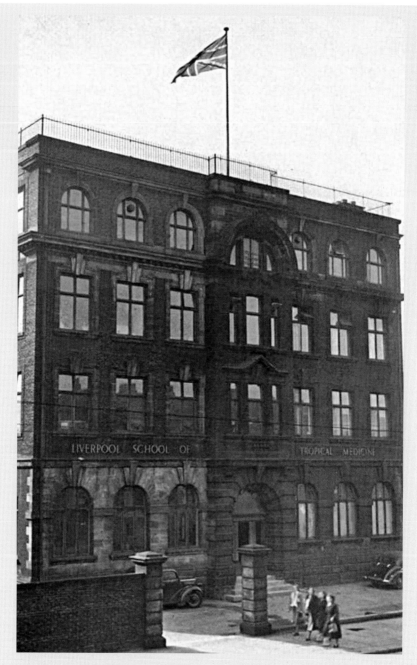

Liverpool School of Tropical Medicine in 1951 – Wikimedia commons for these veterans to undergo Tropical Disease Investigations (TDIs). Far East veterans were often referred by their GPs, or sometimes even self-referred, but the majority of men were sent to Liverpool by the Ministry of Pensions as a result of an application for a war pension. The DHSS funded travel costs and pensions when they were awarded, with the programme becoming big enough to establish a FEPOW Unit- at the DHSS offices in the 1980s. The Tropical School was not an NHS institution, but these men were assessed in NHS beds run by the school and attended to by physicians who were university employed and had honorary NHS Consultant Physician contracts. Many doctors were involved, but the vast majority of TDIs were undertaken by Dr Dion Bell, who saw hundreds of FEPOWs which led to him achieving an iconic status among the FEPOW community. In the 1970s, Dr Geoff Gill (now Emeritus Professor of International Medicine) became involved, mainly in the research side until the last TDI took place in 1999. As well as providing clinical care, LSTM doctors and scientists made advances in laboratory diagnostic tests for conditions such as *Strongyloides stercoralis* (a parasitic infection caused by a nematode worm). They conducted detailed studies into the long-term health effects of Far East captivity and the problems suffered by this group such as chronic neuropathic syndromes, mental health problems and persistent strongyloidiasis.

In more recent years, the LSTM Far East POW project moved to medical historical enquiries into the POW experience, including a major oral history project led by Meg Parkes, in which 67 veterans and 10 wives and widows shared their stories of captivity, survival and the post-war aftermath. Extracts of these interviews and more about Liverpool's FEPOW project can be found here: www.captivememories.org.uk.

My NHS Story

Professor Geoff Gill, Consultant Physician at Aintree University Hospital, and Emeritus Professor of International Medicine at the University of Liverpool reflects on his time in the NHS between 1973 and 2018:

'I qualified in medicine at the University of Newcastle-upon-Tyne and began work for the NHS as a house physician in 1973. Apart from just over three years working abroad, I worked in the NHS continually until finally "hanging up my stethoscope" in early 2018 – a total of 42 years. This included 20 years (1996-2016) as a clinical academic (half university and half NHS), and a few years post-retirement part-time work.

'My leaning was always towards hospital rather than primary care work, and I trained in medicine, becoming a consultant physician (specialising in diabetes and endocrinology) in 1985. The training jobs in those days were house doctor, senior house officer (SHO), registrar, senior registrar and finally consultant. Rotational jobs were only just coming in when I started, and doctors (particularly at SHO level) often took one-off six or 12 month positions. This gave less job security than nowadays but did give some degree of training flexibility. You very much "learnt on the job", and there was nothing like today's system of educational supervisors or on-line training records. However, I do remember that as a senior registrar I met with a regional committee once a year to check on progress and breadth of experience etc. – pretty informal but in some ways more effective than current on-line "box-ticking"!

'The loss of the senior registrar (SR) grade was I think a great shame. This was technically four years but often much longer, and in the medical specialities almost every SR took two years out to do research and write up an MD thesis. Towards the end of the SR grade, you very much acted as a junior consultant. I recall doing a six-month locum consultant physician job in Gateshead in my final SR. Newly appointed consultant physicians in those days were much more able to cope with their new duties and responsibilities.

'Working hours have thankfully reduced from the crazy on-call systems of the 1970s and before. Working weeks of over 100 hours were not uncommon, frequently working a whole day, then on-call for a night, and working the following day also. To be fair, there was much less to do in the way of treatment and investigation, and the number of emergency admissions was significantly smaller than today. We also often covered our own ward only, without emergency "take" duties. Overall, we operated very much as a "firm" with full continuity of care from admission to discharge. Good though this was, I can't see it possible to go back to such a system with the present volume of admissions and limits on junior doctor working hours.

'When I began work in the 1970s, the ward medical system was almost feudal. Consultants were god-like people, with a strict pecking order down the grades below them. Consultant ward rounds were incredibly important affairs, attended by the whole medical firm, and almost always the ward sister. The patient was not expected to make comments or ask questions! In fact, the general lack of patient involvement in those days was quite incredible. Part of this was the culture of the times, and the public were very respectful and deferential to the medical profession. If a diagnosis of cancer was made, patients were often not told, and words like "inflammation" were used. I remember being quite uncomfortable with this practice, though I suspect the patients concerned eventually guessed what was the matter with them.

'The loss of nursing input from our medical ward rounds in recent years has been very regrettable, but overall modern team-based and patient-centred care has been welcome. My later work was mostly on our hospital's Acute Medical Unit, and we were constantly inter-acting with a multitude of healthcare professionals – nurses, pharmacists, physiotherapists, occupational therapists, speech therapists – all on an equal professional basis.

'Politics has to be mentioned, of course, and my career has sadly seen increasing political interference with the running of the NHS from central government. "Reforms" and "consultations" cost a lot of money and rarely improve care. Wheels are constantly being re-invented, and levels of command altered but basic underlying problems remain unanswered – for example overall underfunding, separation of health and social care, and lack of adequately planned workforce numbers.

'Despite all this, some things have not changed. Faced with a sick patient, I have always had the same interaction and communication, using the time honoured skills of history, examination and intervention. And when the assessment was complete, I could do what we physicians should always do: "cure sometimes, help often, support always".'

1970s

The seventies was a decade of strikes – miners, dustmen, postal workers – and financial problems. For most ordinary people, the seventies brought experiences that their grandparents could never have imagined – cheap air travel meant package holidays abroad became commonplace and 91 per cent per cent of people had a (often colour) television. The NHS saw real advances in medical progress. CT scans and transplants became available and the first computers found their way into NHS hospitals. The organisation of the NHS continued to be debated and a new system of Area and Regional health authorities was implemented in 1974 to try to distribute resources more evenly. This was criticized for being too complicated and too top heavy with managers. In the mid-1970s, then health secretary Barbara Castle tried to phase out private patients being treated in NHS facilities. The decade ended with Britain's first female Prime Minister Margaret Thatcher coming into power, and worldwide eradication of smallpox was achieved through vaccination.

1970 **NHS Reorganisation.** The second Green Paper on the NHS rejects the idea of local authorities managing the health service and the debate opens again about the reorganising of the NHS **Conservative government**

1972 **CT Scans introduced.** Computer tomography scans were invented in the late 1960s by Sir Godfrey Hounsfield and became commercially viable in 1972. They revolutionized medical imaging, allowing doctors to see three dimensional views inside the body without performing surgery.
The Cochrane Report sets out the vital importance of randomised controlled trials in assessing the effectiveness of treatments, leading the way for evidence-based medicine

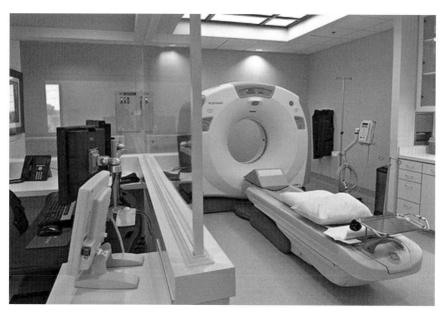

CT Scanner. (Weezie23 via Wikimedia Commons)

The Royal College of General Practitioners is established giving GPs an official representative body

1973   **The NHS Reorganisation Act** (preceded by a 1972 White Paper) sees the traditional tripartite structure replaced in an attempt to generate better co-ordination between health authorities and local authorities. Under the reforms, regional hospital boards are replaced by regional, area and district health authorities, which take over public health and other services (vaccination, health visiting, epidemiological work) from the local authorities. Family planning becomes part of the NHS for the first time. Environmental health and some health education remains a local government responsibility, while the duties of the medical officers for health are transferred to the NHS.

1974   **Labour government**

1975   **The Merrison Report** extends the functions of the GMC (in relation to medical education) to make them more accountable. Disciplinary processes are separated so those whose performances are impaired by ill health are recognized. It is suggested that doctors might undertake some sort of periodic 'relicensure', but the committee decided this was beyond its remit (Revalidation is eventually implemented in 2012 after a series of high profile medical scandals).
        Endorphins are discovered by John Hughes and Hans Kosterlitz at the University of Aberdeen. These polypeptide substances are produced in the brain and resemble opiates in their ability to relieve pain thus working as natural painkillers

1976   **The Resource Allocation Working Party** attempts to address the inequalities between health spending in the south east of England, and the lower levels spent elsewhere. It examines mortality in each area as an indicator of health need and manages from 1977-90 to redistribute resources to the poorer northern regions. 'Cash Limits' are introduced whereby spending authorities cannot exceed the sums of money allocated to them.
        Mandatory training. Three-year postgraduate training programmes for GPs become mandatory

1978   **The world's first IVF baby is born.** Gynaecologist Patrick Steptoe and physiologist Robert Edward develop a technique to fertilize an egg outside the women's body before placing it in the womb, known as in vitro fertilization. Louise Brown is the first 'test tube baby' to be born using this technique. Since then, more than a million children have been born this way worldwide

The Winter of Discontent caused by the oil crisis sees a worsening of the NHS's financial problems

The declaration of Alma Ata calls for urgent action by all governments to protect and promote health. It emphasizes the role of primary care in carrying out public health duties such as immunization, controlling and preventing epidemics, family planning and promoting health and nutrition.

1979   **First Bone marrow transplant** is performed on a child with primary immunodeficiency at Great Ormond Street Hospital by Professor Roland Levinsky. Bone marrow helps create the body's immune system and today, the Antony Nolan Trust recruits bone marrow donors for those who suffer with diseases such as leukaemia and non-Hodgkins lymphoma.

Wearing seat belts made compulsory for drivers and front seat passengers in a car.

Conservative government

Council house tenants given the right to buy their own home.

My NHS Story

Sister Judith Susser started her State Registered Nurse training at the Manchester Royal Infirmary (MRI) in 1972 and continued working in the NHS until recently. She shares her thoughts on her 45 year career:

'In retrospect I was very naive when I started my training and not politically minded so I therefore took the NHS for granted and never gave the organisation a second thought – I just wanted to survive from placement to placement and qualify.

'In brief, I qualified and worked as a staff nurse at MRI for 6 months, then went to Israel for 1 year as a volunteer nurse working in Beer Sheva in their (rudimentary) ITU. On return to the UK I worked privately in The Convent Nursing Home in Nottingham before going to

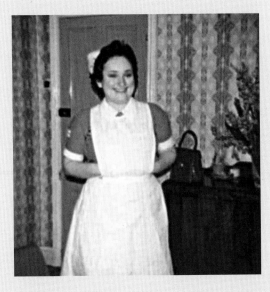

do a Urology and Nephrology course at The 3 P's [Footnote - The three P's is the name given to the hospital group comprised of St Phillip's, St Peter's and St Paul's – which closed in 1992] in London. I worked there from 1977, moving to the Middlesex Hospital, then UCLH.

'For the last 15 years I have worked on the Spinal Cord Injury Centre at the Royal National Orthopaedic Hospital in Stanmore. In this specialised rehabilitation setting I am proud to say that there is total holistic care involving rehabilitation physicians, surgeons, neuro-physiologists, physios, OTs, dieticians, psychologists, psychiatrists, tissue viability teams, speech and language specialists, community liaison workers, fertility specialists, urologists and bowel care teams. The patients are with us from 3 months to 1 year and remain under our care for the rest of their lives. THIS is the NHS at its finest.

'I was so young and simple when I started at MRI. I had never seen anyone naked, or drunk, or indeed both at the same time! I was totally impressionable, and in awe of anyone senior to me, which was everyone. Terrifyingly I don't recall being phased by my total lack of knowledge, and I never questioned or queried anything. Questioning was not then in my nature, and I suspect it was not encouraged. Donning the complicated uniform gave me the confidence to face the world, but I was probably a total liability.

'After an introductory 6-8 weeks we were let loose on the wards. There was a lot of bed-making, bed baths, bedpan and urinal "rounds".

When patients returned from the operating theatre, after an hour or so they had a "post-op" wash. This comprised washing hands and face with a flannel, checking the dressings, swapping theatre gown for a nightie, changing the draw sheet and giving a mouth wash. The draw sheet was about one yard wide and was placed over a rubber sheet, (later to be superseded by plastic) under the patient's bottom. This was to save the necessity of changing the bottom bed sheet, probably not ideal for tissue viability.... all those potential creases and wrinkles. I believe the post-op wash does not exist anymore as so many procedures are now day cases. Nevertheless, it "freshened up" the patient, allowed assessment of their pain and general condition, and was an excellent example of old fashioned bedside care, that was most likely very welcome.

'Tasks were allocated as "rounds" to be completed. The "back" round involved taking a trolley from bed to bed giving pressure area care. Some patients were in bed for many days, but I do not remember seeing any pressure sores, so this must have been effective. My favourite round, being of an organised disposition, was "Obs". Again, with a trolley I went from bed to bed taking patient observations and completing their charts. Similarly, and just as enjoyable was doing the fluid In and Out charts. My charts were impeccable, but I'm ashamed to say I had no critical evaluation faculties, therefore a patient may have been haemorrhaging internally or seriously dehydrated and no alarm bells rang in my task driven skull.

'The first Christmas I experienced was lovely. The hospital was made up of long, narrow Nightingale wards. We were asked to sit with elderly patients, at their bedside. A choir of nurses led by the sisters, with their navy, red-lined capes worn inside-out, and carrying lanterns sang walking from ward to ward, the lights being dimmed. I remember with moving anticipation hearing the choir move from ward to ward.

'There was unfortunately some, what would now constitute institutional bullying. Looking back, the first bed-bath I was asked to perform alone was on an elderly male patient. I was told to wash, dress him and get him up. When I went behind the screens there was a prosthetic leg leaning up against the wall. My face must have been a picture! Then there was being sent to the stores department for both a "long stand" and a "dead weight". It surprises me that I'm not still stupidly standing there!

'We were in charge on night duty probably after 1 year in training. We worked with one or two nursing auxiliaries and were supervised by the night sister who covered many wards. I do not recall being aghast at this huge responsibility, as I would be now. Ah, the callowness of youth. I do remember the satisfaction of doing the late night drink round, Ovaltine or Horlicks, maybe a Mackeson, closing the blinds and dimming the lights and settling the patients down to sleep.

'One morning, as a staff nurse, I was giving out breakfast on my ward, which had been divided into 6 bed bays. I trundled my trolley round calling to the patients "porridge or flakes, hot milk or cold, sugar, tea or coffee?" One patient lay sleeping. I yelled these choices a couple of times, the other patients watching me. Eventually it dawned on me that he was not going to need breakfast that day, or ever again. I pulled the curtains round the bed and tried to compose my face prior to walking out past five pairs of knowing eyes.

'Nowadays, watching programmes such as 24 Hours in A&E, I say: "Thank God for the NHS." It seems to me that the more over-managed and beleaguered it becomes, the more these programmes proliferate. In my area of North Central London an external focus group gathered views and trends within the nursing workforce. They found a lack of new and younger staff climbing the ranks, and that among the nurses over 50 years of age, the majority were sticking around for financial reasons, rather than the joy of the job.

'I handed in my notice to retire, after another demeaning interaction with manager, who wanted us to move office again in a reorganisation that made no sense, then said to me in a meeting, when I queried this, "I'm not asking you, I'm telling you." I still do my old job for two days a week on the "bank", until they advertise and fill my position, predictably at a lower grade.'

1980s

The eighties are remembered for big hair and shoulder pads, and the emergence of a frightening new disease – AIDS – which caused previous healthy people to die from rare conditions. The AIDS epidemic began in 1981, when unusual clusters of pneumocystis pneumonia were reported in homosexual men in Los Angeles. Homophobia was rife, and the disease was initially labelled GRID (Gay Related Immune Deficiency) until it was evident that half of those affected were not homosexual. The disease was poorly understood, and millions died until HIV was discovered as the cause and developments in immunology meant treatments started to become available. The eighties saw a rise in drug resistance – widespread use of antibiotics since the 1940s had allowed infectious organisms to adapt to become resistant, meaning the drugs used to kill them were no longer effective. There was a focus on preventative medicine in the eighties and a notion that individuals were responsible for their own health and lifestyle choices and breast and cervical screening programs were introduced to the NHS. Privatisation took off in the eighties – with British Telecom, British Gas, British Steel and the Water Authorities (among others) all being affected. British Rail followed in the nineties. The NHS looked like it would follow suit when Margaret Thatcher announced plans to reform the NHS and introduce an internal market.

1980   **MRI (Magnetic Resonance Imaging) Scans** are introduced providing detailed information about the soft tissues of the body by using a combination of magnetism and radio frequency waves.
        Laparoscopic (Keyhole) Surgery is used for the first time to remove a gallbladder.

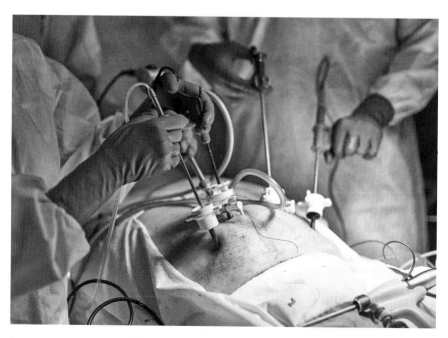

Laparoscopy operation. (Abode Stock Images)

The Black Report, commissioned by the Labour Government in 1977, investigates inequalities in health, finding that those in lower socioeconomic groups suffer higher rates of mortality. Access to health services, particularly preventative services is poor among the working class. It recommends increased spending on community health and primary care, and government intervention with increased child benefits, improved housing and agreeing minimum working conditions with unions. The new conservative government did not endorse these recommendations due to the scale of expenditure involved.

1981   **First UK death from AIDS**. A 41-year-old man dies from an acquired immunodeficiency syndrome (AIDS) related illness in London. Terry Higgins was one of the first people to die of the disease a year later, leading to the formation of the Terrance Higgins Trust. By 1984, scientists had identified that human immunodeficiency virus (HIV) caused AIDS and testing was introduced in 1985. The 'Don't die of ignorance' public health campaign was launched in 1987. Triple combination therapy

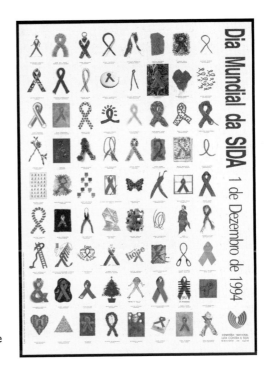

World AIDS Day 1994. (Wellcome Collection)

(Highly active anti-retroviral therapy or HAART) became standard in 1996 and HIV treatment became free for everyone in England in 2012. The term AIDS describes a set of illnesses people with HIV can get if they don't receive treatment. In the 1980s, HIV treatment wasn't so good and most people would eventually succumb to these diseases. Today, treatment is so good that few people develop AIDS. People newly diagnosed with HIV today can expect a normal life expectancy, if they have timely diagnosis and treatment. The landmark PARTNER study recently showed that people with HIV who are on effective treatment to suppress their viral load, cannot pass HIV on to others. In August 2017, NHS England started a trial of HIV prevention drugs (Pre-exposure prophylaxis or PrEP) to people at high risk of HIV infection.

1982   **NHS Reorganisation** – the area tier of NHS management is abolished resulting in the creation of 192 district health authorities (DHAs) that are responsible to the regional health authorities with the aim of simplifying the structure. This is the start of many more re-organisations over the next 3 decades **National Confidential Enquiry into Patient Outcome and Death (NCEPOD)** is born. A review of surgical and anaesthetic practice is reviewed over a year in 1982, known as the Confidential Enquiry into Peri-Operative Deaths (CEPOD). The venture is given government funding and renamed NCEPOD in 1988, extending its remit to include medical patients in 2002. Today, NCEPOD is an independent charity that reviews patient care by undertaking confidential surveys and research. NCEPOD reports have shaped the way healthcare is delivered in the UK, and their recommendations have created good practices such as peer review of mortality after surgery and ensuring hospitals admitting emergency patients have access to 24-hour radiology, operating and recovery rooms.

1983   **The Mental Health Act** introduces the issue of consent to treatment. Prior to this, a detained patient could be treated against their will, even if they were a 'voluntary' patient. The mental health act allows people to be detained (or 'sectioned') against their will for the urgent treatment of mental disorders if they are at risk of harm to themselves or others.

The Griffiths report is published, heralding a new managerial age in the NHS. It advocates NHS management boards at arm's length from the government, and general managers with responsibility for performance and budgets in hospitals and district health authorities, bringing their experiences of business school and the private sector to NHs leadership. Doctors are encouraged to become involved with corporate decision making

The UKCC (United Kingdom Central Council for Nursing, Midwifery and Health Visiting) is set up to replace the General Nursing Council in maintaining a register of nurses

1986   **First case of BSE in cattle** is reported by the State Veterinary Service in the UK. Bovine Spongiform encephalopathy or 'Mad Cow Disease' caused fatal changes to the brains of cows. In 1990, a domestic cat was diagnosed with the disease, raising concerns that transmission to humans was possible. Up until 1996, when the link is acknowledged, the government told the public there was no evidence the disease could be passed onto humans. An estimated 400,000 cattle infected with BSE entered the food chain in the 1980s, and over the next 25 years, 177 people contracted and died from a disease with similar neurological symptoms called new variant Creutzfeldt-Jakob disease (vCJD) thought to be from eating contaminated beef. Mass slaughter of infected herds takes place and a ban on exporting British Beef is imposed by the European Union. The BSE enquiry is published in 2000 and concludes that the crisis was a result of intensive farming and cows being fed with dead animal remains. The government's reassurance campaign was branded a mistake which left the public feeling betrayed. Chernobyl nuclear disaster

1987   **Promoting Better Health** – The government's plans for improving health are published in this White Paper, pledging a fee for primary care doctors taking part in health promotion work such as health checks and immunisations. These proposals formed the basis of the 1990 GP contracts

The world's first heart, liver and lung transplant takes place in Cambridge at Papworth hospital, carried out by Professor Sir Roy Calne and Professor John Wallwork. The patient survives ten years and her healthy heart is then donated to another transplant patient.

1988 **National cervical screening** introduced. Screening is the process of identifying individuals who appear healthy but may be at increased risk of a condition. It is an imperfect process and in every screen there can be false positive and false negative results. Cervical screening aims to prevent cervical cancer by detecting and treating abnormalities of the cervix. Today, Liquid based cytology (LBC) is used to collect samples of cells from the cervix. Currently in England it is available to women aged between 25-64. Human Papilloma virus (HPV) is a common virus transmitted usually through sexual contact, which will be cleared by the immune system in the same way it would fight the common cold. There are over a 100 subtypes of this virus, and some high risk subtypes (HR-HPV) have been linked with the development of abnormal cervical cells – which left untreated, may go on to develop into cervical cancer. If cell changes are detected and HR-HPV is present, then women will be referred for colposcopy, where the cervix can be viewed under a microscope to determine if further treatment is required.

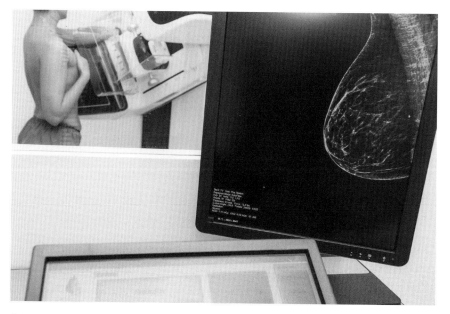

A mammogram. (Abobe Stock Images)

Measles, mumps, rubella (MMR) vaccine introduced

Breast screening introduced. The Forrest report on breast cancer screening concluded there was a convincing case to screen women over the age of 50 with mammograms (x-rays of the breasts), as long as there would be effective resources in place to deal with any abnormalities found through the process. **Routine newborn hearing testing** is introduced at Whipps Cross University Hospital using otoacoustic emission technology

Lockerbie bombing

1989 **Working for Patients** – the government's White Paper sets out plans to reform the NHS, introducing the creation of the internal market by splitting the bodies that provide care from those that purchase it. Health authorities are required to manage their own budgets to purchase the best possible healthcare services for their areas – even if that means favouring external organisations over their own local hospitals. Meanwhile, hospitals can apply to become NHS trusts – independent organisations with their own management. GPs with registered populations of at least 11,000 patients, are able to apply for practice budgets to purchase hospital services.

Project 2000 is implemented following the Judge report of 1985, which recommended the transfer of nurse training to Universities. Concerns are raised regarding acquisition of practical as well as academic skills

Fall of the Berlin wall

My NHS Story

Dr David Wingfield is a senior partner at Brook Green Medical Centre in Hammersmith, and chairman of the Hammersmith and Fulham GP Federation. He reflects on his 30 years working in the NHS.

'As with many doctors, I suppose, I took my decision to specialise, in General practice, because of the inspiration of another. My teacher David El Kabir demonstrated personal commitment to the people of Notting Hill building up his registered patient list from nothing and

81

in so doing generated huge mutual commitment, the foundation of the relationship between doctor and patient.

'He inspired us, as his students, to found a charity for the homeless of central London, Wytham Hall, where we could care for them when sick and unable to endure the terrible hardships of life on the street. I entered the world of General Practice therefore assuming that a career founded on a vocation and public service was at the heart of the NHS. What a surprise was in store.

'One of my first awakenings was a conference on Single Homelessness in London where a report was launched and purported to offer solutions to an age-old problem. It was nothing of the kind. Where the SHIL report offered numerical analysis and quantities it had no depth of understanding. What it asked for was political shift but the direction was unclear because its whole analysis was superficial. While this report is now long confined to the history books the cycle of reports offering analysis, understanding and solutions has continued unabated.

'The GP was always the poor relation of doctors in the NHS hierarchy of specialties. Competition between doctors to the point of aggression was commonplace and horrified many of us who had to endure consultants behaving like demigods. Why I wondered was this tolerated in a National Health Service that was supposed to deliver care to all patients equally and from cradle to grave? The focus on the patient and holistic practice was it seemed to me understood to be a matter for the Nursing profession and the GP. After the foundation of the Royal College of GPs in 1952 these principles were enshrined in statute and seemed at least for a while to assure the foundations and purpose of the field I was committed to work within.

'When I was starting out as a GP it was thought that the NHS could be run more professionally and efficiently if a professional managerial element was introduced. The influential Griffiths report (1983) ushered in this imaginative new dynamic but as Brian Jarman subsequently lamented in a BMJ editorial some 30 years later, managers remained in a fundamentally different place from clinical leaders and rather than complementing clinical leadership, management tried over time to control it. This has contributed to the current state whereby doctors at all levels of the NHS are disillusioned and confused by perceived controls over their clinical autonomy. Clinical leadership is now being reinvented, albeit in a straitjacket of guidelines and policies.

'Looking back over a career of over 30 years I see that key elements of the NHS have struggled to change.

'Firstly, a misunderstanding of what is required when confronted with a balance of risk. A limited analysis has too often been coupled with the reversion to bureaucratic processes and appeal to hierarchy when confronting difficult problems. "It was someone else's decision". "I had no ability to control or take the decision". I often now ask who is in charge only to find that no-one is able to answer. Take as an example the programme of planned hospital closures in North West London. There is no evidence that fewer hospital beds will be achievable and even less that there is a systematic programme of replacement with community resources at a very much greater scale from hitherto. Central London Hospitals on Red Alert with no beds is now sadly commonplace, even in summer.

'Secondly, an undue emphasis on a Public Health or "population" viewpoint which, though it has many merits, does undermine the very personal relationship between the doctor and the patient. What is good for the many is not necessarily right for the individual. The widespread and increasing use of statin medications is a case in point here. Many patients stand to gain from such treatment and the scientific basis is strong. But prescribing based on target populations and control of cholesterol levels to change outcomes for society is wrong thinking at the level of the individual who may wish to make different and more personal decisions.

'The beginnings of professional accountability are emerging in the form of integrated services across primary and secondary care, hospital and community services, nurses and doctors. GPs nationwide are hearing the call to arms and forming organisations that offer the possibility of primary care services at scale (whether through large partnerships or federations of various forms). Given their head they may yet prove that the NHS has a future. But shackled with senseless financial rules and contractual procedures (often distanced from outcomes) from an unaccountable managerial system one can but recall William Blake who wrote: "Bound and weary I thought best, to sulk upon my mother's breast".

'I look forward to an NHS which continues to deliver its founding principles, but I am not optimistic. The cracks are already emerging in the form of short-term solutions, outsourced services with poor contractual managerial control, and worst of all a financing system which is set on affordability rather than with regard to the expectations of the service to deliver. NHS professionalized management has now had over 20 years to prove itself. It has not done so and should be reformed along with a return to a patient focused professionally led NHS with doctors playing a prominent part. Our patients (and I count myself in their number) will not forgive us if we let them down.'

1990s

The nineties saw increasing choices for patients and the creation of services such as NHS Direct. Advances in technology and the rise of the internet shaped society, leading to the emergence of expert patients and multiple health charities. The Human Genome project took off and gene therapy developed, as did cloning and the use of human tissue in medicine, while the MMR Scandal and GP serial killer Harold Shipman hit the headlines. The concept of Commissioning was introduced to the NHS in the early 1990s, when the 'internal market' was born – internal, because both buyers and sellers of services were NHS organisations. Commissioning is the process of planning, securing and monitoring services and until 1989, health authorities decided on the amount of care needed and provided it through their own hospitals. The Conservative government introduced these market theories into healthcare, on the premise that the public sector is inefficient, and the private sector brings growth and innovation. They argued that by making providers compete for resources, greater efficiency and innovation would be encouraged. When Labour came into power in 1997, they fiercely opposed the internal market, and abolished GP Fundholding … only to reverse their position and re-introduce it under a new name a few years later (Practice Based Commissioning). Labour also devolved power to an elected parliament in Scotland and an elected assembly in Wales and Northern Ireland, resulting in four separate health systems.

1990 NHS reorganisation – The National Health Service Community Care Act receives Royal assent, pushing through the proposals of the 1989 Working for Patients paper to split the provision and purchasing (or commissioning) of healthcare. The act allowed the Secretary of State for Health to establish NHS trusts by order. The trusts assumed responsibility for the ownership and management of hospitals that were previously managed by the regional or district health authorities.

New GP contracts saw greater external management of general practice and established financial incentives for GPs to become more involved in health promotion activity. GPs received payment for collating information such as the height, weight and blood pressure of patients. GP fundholding allowed GPs to take on responsibilities for commissioning services for patients, becoming more involved with the wider health system. Not all GPs become fundholders, and those who do not have services purchased for them by the local health authorities. This brings criticism that a two-tier system has been created, in which patients in practices with GP Fundholders are able to access care more rapidly.

NHS Confederation is founded (initially as the National Association of Health Authorities and Trusts) as a membership body for NHS organisations. Members include acute and foundation trusts, community health service providers, mental health service providers, ambulance trusts and clinical commissioning groups. It claims to represent the whole NHS and runs an annual conference for senior decision makers.

Poll tax riots

1991   **The Patients' Charter** is first published, setting out patients' rights within the NHS and the service they can expect to receive. The charter sets out targets for waiting times for hospital treatment

        The Gulf War

1992   **The Health of the Nation** White Paper is published and identifies coronary heart disease, cancer, mental health, HIV care, sexual health and accidents as areas for improvement. There is an emphasis on individual responsibility for health

        The Internet starts to take off in the UK as dial up internet access is introduced

1994   **The NHS Organ Donor Register** is set up following a campaign by parents John and Rosemary Cox, whose son Peter died of a brain tumour and wanted to donate his organs to help others.

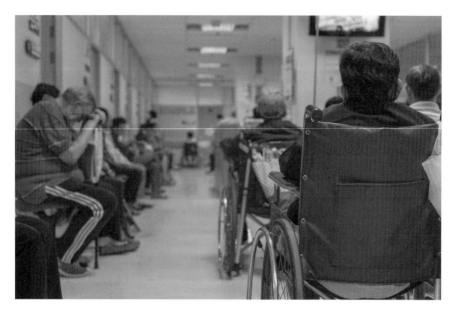

Patient's waiting for care. (Adobe Stock Images)

NHS Reorganisation – the number of regional health authorities is reduced to eight
The Channel Tunnel opens

1996   **National Screening Committee established**

1997   **Labour government**
The New NHS: Modern, Dependable is a White Paper produced by the new Labour government which leads to further NHS reorganisation. It aims to replace the internal market with a more integrated system, but still retains the purchaser-provider split introduced by the conservatives. GP Fundholding is abolished due to concerns of a two-tier system.
Dolly the sheep – first mammalian clone

1998   **MMR Scandal begins** with the publication of a paper by Dr Andrew Wakefield in the *Lancet* suggesting a link between the MMR (Measles, Mumps, Rubella) vaccination and autism. Parents across the world avoid vaccinating their children due to a fear of autism. Measles outbreaks and deaths in 2008 and 2009 are attributed to not vaccinating. Scientists published many more studies proving no link. Wakefield is investigated and found to be guilty of deliberate fraud and is struck off the medical register. His study was funded by anti-vaccine lawyers and found to be full of ethical violations. He picked data that supported his argument and ignored data that didn't, and he deliberately falsified facts for financial gain. The *Lancet* subsequently withdrew his paper.

The National Institute for Clinical Excellence (NICE) and the Commission for health improvement is established as a special health authority to provide national guidance on quality and reduce variation in the availability and quality of NHS treatments – the so-called postcode lottery. NICE is responsible for producing national evidence-based guidance on health promotion, health technologies, social care and disease treatment and prevention. They also develop quality standards for those providing and commissioning services. (NICE is also responsible for developing QOF – the Quality Outcomes Framework – a voluntary incentive scheme for all GP practices in the UK, which rewards them financially

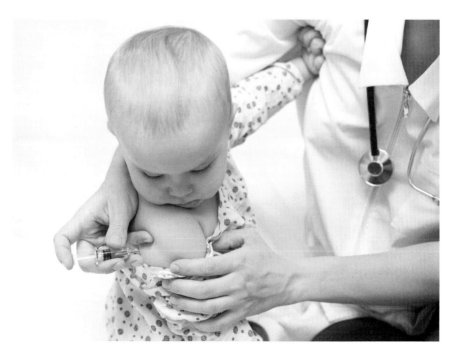

(Adobe Stock Images)

for how well they care for patients. Under the scheme, GP practices score points according to their level of achievement against a series of indicators, such as the percentage of patients with a new diagnosis of a disease who are referred for certain tests. As part of the Health and Social Care Act 2012, NICE became established in legislation as a Non-Departmental Public Body (NDPB) accountable to the Department of Health, but operationally independent. NICE attempts to assess the cost effectiveness of NHS expenditures to determine whether or not they represent value for money. New treatments are analysed relative to the next best treatment currently in use using Quality-Adjusted Life Years (QALY) to quantify the expected health benefits.

NHS Direct is set up as a 24 hour telephone advice line staffed by nurses, aiming to provide people with fast advice and information about health and NHS services at home. This closed in 2014 due to financial problems and was replaced by NHS 111, an 'urgent but not life threatening' advice line staffed by telephone operators, to complement the long running 999 emergency number. 999 is the world's oldest emergency telephone number and was introduced to London in 1937 after a house fire killed five women. An outraged neighbour complained she had been kept on hold when trying to contact the local fire brigade, and 999 was born.

The European Working Time Directive (EWTD) takes effect in UK law in October 1998 to protect the health and safety of workers in the European Union. It dictates minimum requirements regarding working hours, annual leave and rest periods. Doctors in training were exempt from the EWTD until August 2004. Its implementation was examined in a report commissioned by Medical Education England (now Health Education England) which found it had impacted training opportunities.

1999 **NHS Reorganisation.** After the abolition of GP Fundholding, 481 Primary Care Groups are created to replace it – technically subcommittees of the District Health Authorities. These later become Primary Care Trusts in 2000. A *BMJ* editorial comments that this reorganisation is 'universalizing fundholding, while repudiating the concept'.
The Euro is introduced.

My NHS Story

Lianna Brinded is a Journalist and Broadcaster who shares her view that the NHS is broken and needs fixing now.

'The NHS is the jewel in the crown for Britain. Whoever you are, wherever you are, you can count on having a doctor or a nurse see to you for free. Well, when we mean free, funded by the taxpayer. Countries like the US have such a chronically expensive, complicated, and discriminatory system that if you're poor, you have to really weigh up whether you are able to afford those stitches because you fell over in the street, have that baby, or even potentially life-saving medication for your long-term illness. So, in comparison, the NHS looks like a dream.

'But this is a dangerous way of thinking. The NHS was probably fit for purpose 60 years ago but our society is larger, more diverse, and complex and the model that once was the saviour for the masses can now be an active hindrance for care.

'Our social media feeds are awash of people being grateful for the treatment they have or didn't have. It's full of stories of not being seen on time, being denied scans or treatment, or being told we're wasting NHS time. But you still have people peddling out this "but at least we have the NHS."

'The issue is that we are a nation of reactionary medicine and care, not preventative. The whole system runs on trying to fix things when it's too late rather than do the necessary scans, treatment, or care in the first place that would prevent long-term problems, pain, heartache, and death. When the NHS screws up, people are in pain, their livelihoods ruined, or even die.

'My family, like many others, is littered with stories of NHS horrors. My father, a previously healthy person, suddenly blacked out and had a fit. The hospital just said he was stressed and refused to give him even one scan. Turns out a year later he had a brain tumour sitting on his optic nerve that had grown rapidly in that one year. What happened next was a year of systematic bad care, mistakes, and corner cutting that helped accelerate his death. He wasn't even 50.

'My mother had a mild stroke in the middle of the restaurant that was conveniently located next door to one of London's top hospitals.

The paramedics came and didn't take her across the road for treatment. I urged and begged for her to get seen to—they wouldn't budge. The whole episode was even more distressing considering this is how my father was allowed to incubate a tumour that could've been dealt with had the doctors and other staff done the logical thing and given scans. It's even more sickening that my mum was a NHS nurse for decades and she couldn't even get the care when she needed it.

'Friends who have broken their legs, wrists, ankles, have been taken to hospital only to not even be given scans or treatment. Many have been left with problems that have resulted in corrective surgery years down the line or life-long mobility issues because they didn't get the right care in the first place. I know people who were incapable of breathing properly and diagnosed with asthma because it was easy to, in lieu of doing any investigations—turns out they were being strangled from the inside by abnormal growths.

'These tales aren't just isolated horror stories, they are part and parcel of the system we have today. But we can't blame the government of not spending—it's risen every year. It's about how the NHS uses it, which is a responsibility for the sector as well as people who use it.

'We have some of the worst availability of beds in hospitals, we waste over £1 billion a year in missed appointments—and nearly the same amount has been wasted on a failed IT system. We quibble over giving an expensive scan to someone in the first stage, yet spend thousands more per person to fix something that could've been prevented. We have some of the worst cancer survival rates in Europe and parts of the developed world because we hold back on using certain drugs or giving the relevant treatment in the first place. There are campaigns telling us not to go to doctors for various things, even though that cough could be something sinister and could end up being an ailment that could kill the very young, old, or vulnerable.

'It's not just a structural change that's needed—it's an attitude change. For a "free" service, of course we'll always feel under-funded, under-staffed. But then would everyone be willing to pay more out of their taxes? Tax hikes are deeply unpopular.

'Changing the NHS to a prevention service from a reactionary one will be hard but it's something that former health secretaries, doctors, and key NHS officials have been asking for. Not only will it make the whole system more efficient, it will also mean we use the money in the right way to give the care and treatment we all deserve.'

2000s

The new millennium brings with it further NHS reshuffling and financial crises. New Labour's victory in 1997 brought the NHS Plan in 2000 which promised to rebuild the NHS for the twenty-first century. PFIs, PCTS and foundation trusts are born and the four hour target is introduced to emergency departments. Terrorism shocks the world with attacks in New York, Spain and closer to home in London. There is an influx of migrants, particularly from the European Union and retired Brits also emigrate to sunnier climes in their thousands, prompting the government to say that the NHS should not be free for those who do not live in the UK. Smoking is banned in public places in 2007 and smart phones and social media become commonplace by the end of the decade. The NHS tries to keep up by introducing the National Programme for IT, aiming for a paperless NHS. Its ultimate failure is deemed to be a result of an underestimation of the scale of the project, combined with a top down management approach – centralized authority making decisions on behalf of local organisations, with a lack of adequate engagement with the people actually using it.

2000   **NHS Plan** sets out a strategy to increase staffing, hospital beds and decrease waiting times. This is formalized by the 2001 Health and Social Care Act. A new model of financing is agreed called the **Private Finance Initiative (PFI)**, which involves using private sector money instead of public money. Loans are taken from private companies with high interest rates (some over 70 per cent per cent) to build new hospitals and clinics, which the NHS is required to pay off like a mortgage over the following decades. These schemes are poorly negotiated by civil servants against opportunistic financiers resulting in huge debts for NHS trusts. A report from the Centre for Health and the Public interest in 2017 showed that companies running PFI contracts between 2010-2015, to build and run NHS hospitals and services made pre-tax profits of £831m from the NHS– money which has been taken away from patient care and is often more than it cost to build the hospitals in the first place. Over the next five years, £1bn of taxpayers funds will go towards paying for PFIs.

NHS Walk in Centres open to deal with minor illnesses and injuries offering round the clock access. They are nurse led, available to everyone without needing an appointment or needing to register.

2001   **Bristol Heart Scandal** report published. During the 1990s, high mortality rates were found among babies undergoing cardiac surgery at the Bristol Royal Infirmary. The inquiry revealed a lax approach to safety, with a lack of leadership, teamwork and staff shortages, which ultimately led to the development of regulatory bodies (see below).

The Commission for Healthcare Improvement is created, as directed by the Health Act of 1999. This is the first organization to formally assess the performance of NHS hospitals (now known as the Care Quality Commission or CQC)

The National Patient Safety Agency is set up (now part of NHS Improvement) to drive improved patient care, prompted by reports such as the DoH's report 'An Organization with a Memory' which suggested that every year, 28,000 written complaints are made about aspects of clinical treatment in NHS hospitals; that hospital-acquired infections cost the NHS £1billion and that over £400million is paid by the NHS annually to settle clinical negligence claims.

9-11 Terrorist Attack on the World Trade centre

2002   **NHS Reorganisations.** Based on the White Paper 'Shifting the balance of power', 95 Health authorities are abolished and partly replaced by **Primary Care Trusts (PCTs)** which are set up as administrative bodies, responsible for commissioning healthcare, and 28 strategic health authorities, which are to provide regional management for the NHS and oversee the PCTs. The PCTs are given responsibility for 80 per cent per cent of the health budget.

The Nursing and Midwifery Council (NMC) is founded to regulate nurses and midwives and set educational standards, replacing the UKCC.

National Programme for IT (NPfIT) is launched with the idea of creating a paperless NHS, with an integrated IT system throughout the entire NHS (30,000 GPs and 300 hospitals). An agency called NHS Connecting for Health was formed in

2005 to deliver this project (replacing what was before it – the NHS Information Authority). The motivation for the ambitious project came from Cabinet level, but the delivery did not translate into reality. Hit by technical problems and contractual wrangling, the £11bn scheme was scrapped in 2011 and labelled a fiasco. The Health and Social Care Information centre (HSCIC) was created as a special health authority and took over parts of the NPfIT in 2013 when NHS Connecting for Health ceased to exist. It was rebranded as the catchier NHS Digital in 2016. NHS Digital now runs the Spine service in England – a central, secure system for patient data. This comprises the Electronic Prescription service, which sends prescriptions digitally from GPs to pharmacies; The Summary Care Record-which allows authorized NHS staff to see important clinical information about patients to provide the best care; the e-referral service which manages the booking of hospital appointments; the Child Protection information sharing service which helps collate safeguarding concerns.

The Wanless Report, commissioned by the Treasury to look at healthcare spending and future trends, concluded that future NHS spending would rise, mainly due to patients demanding more choice and higher quality services. The author recommended spending more on IT and enhancing the role of primary care.

2003   **NHS Reorganisation**. The Health and Social care (Community Standards) Act is passed, allowing for the establishment of foundation trusts and new GP contracts. This act introduced 'Alternate Provider Medical Services' or APMS contracts, which allowed non-NHS providers to be commissioned by the PCTs to deliver care.

Foundation Trusts are established as part of the government's plan to continue the internal market. There are set up as a 'halfway house' between the public and private sectors to try to make healthcare more efficient. Foundation status aims to give trust managers financial and managerial freedom from the Department of Health, by allowing them to borrow money privately, without prior approval from the Treasury, and invest this money as they see fit in local services

Monitor is established to regulate NHS foundation trusts in terms of quality and finances. It became part of NHS Improvement in 2016

Independent Sector Treatment Centres (ISTC) are first opened. These centers focus on providing routine elective treatments, (such as cataract surgery) for NHS patients by the private sector as part of the 2000 NHS Plan to reduce NHS waiting lists, promising greater efficiency and patient choice. They promised more than they delivered. Unable to employ NHS staff at the outset, they were staffed by overseas doctors, whose quality of training and familiarity with the NHS was questioned. They negatively impacted the training of junior doctors, who previously learned by doing the 'straightforward' procedures the ISTCs took on. The finances were also problematic, in that they were paid whether they reached the required targets or not. They were not regulated in the same way as the NHS, and data could not be collected on their productivity in the same way as in the NHS due to commercial sensitivity and poor data collection.

Tobacco Adverts banned

2004   **New GP contracts** are renegotiated, resulting in more autonomy for practices regarding the range of services they provide and a focus on performance related pay for reaching standards set out in the Quality and Outcomes Framework (QOF). Stronger regulatory mechanisms are introduced for GPs including annual appraisals and a requirement to register with the CQC. GPs traditionally carried out evening house calls and emergency night visits providing continuity to their patients. The new contracts allowed GPs to opt out of this (virtually all did) passing responsibility for out of hours care to the PCTs. Private companies (such as Harmoni, Serco and Virgin) stepped in to take this role costing more than 392 million in 2005. Hospital consultant's contracts are also re-negotiated, aiming to increase the direct amount of time they spend with patients.

Four hour targets are introduced into emergency departments to reduce waiting times. The NHS Plan in 2000 stated that by 2004, no-one should be waiting for more than four hours in the emergency department from arrival to admission, transfer or discharge, and financial incentives to meet these targets were introduced. Government funding was invested in recruiting new ED nurses increasing consultant numbers. New strategies were introduced to achieve these targets and improve patient flow. Emergency Nurse Practitioners (ENPs) assessed and treated patients with minor injuries to avoid the wait to see a doctor, and money was invested in other NHS services – such as NHS Direct and GP out of hours care. Waiting times did reduce, however reports of compromised patient care due to management pressures to meet the targets were notably reported in the Mid Staffs enquiry. Targets are a way for the government to focus the entire NHS on a priority, which they can then show to voters and taxpayers to explain what their money is achieving.

Agenda for change (AfC) comes into operation, and remains the grading and pay system used for staff in the NHS (with the exception of doctors, dentists and some managers). It allocates posts to set paybands to try to evaluate the job rather than the person doing it, to create uniformity across the NHS.

Facebook launched

Boxing Day Tsunami An earthquake in the Indian Ocean on Boxing Day is the third largest earthquake ever recorded triggering a series of tsunamis throughout Asia. It is one of the deadliest natural disasters in recorded history

2005   **The Shipman Inquiry is closed.** GP and serial killer Harold Shipman shattered the faith in the medical profession after he was exposed as a serial killer, responsible for the deaths of up to 215 patients. The inquiry started after his trial in 2000, with the final report being release in 2005. Shipman was jailed for life for murdering fifteen of his patients, and subsequently committed suicide in jail. An array of changes were introduced following the inquiry, including changes to the death certification process, safer management of controlled drugs and monitoring of prescribing data, systems to monitor mortality rates and unexpected deaths, revalidation and appraisal of GPs and GP practice inspections.

London Terrorist bombings

Modernising Medical Careers (MMC) replaced the traditional training grades in postgraduate medical education. The traditional first year Pre-Registration House Officer (PRHO)

and first year Senior House Officer (SHO) grades were replaced by a 2 year Foundation Programme (Foundation House Officer 1 and 2, or F1 and F2). Further speciality training replaced the old Specialist Registrar (SpR) grade, with trainees being awarded a certificate of completion of training (CCT) and entry to the specialist or GP register at the end of training. MMC was part of the NHS Plan 2000 which aimed to increase consultant numbers by 'modernising the SHO grade' or reducing the amount of training time doctors undertake before they become consultants. The old system allowed doctors the flexibility to try a variety of different jobs and gain valuable experience before deciding what to specialize in. The transition to the new system was disastrous. The Postgraduate Medical Education and Training Board initially recruited centrally, resulting in thousands of doctors being left without

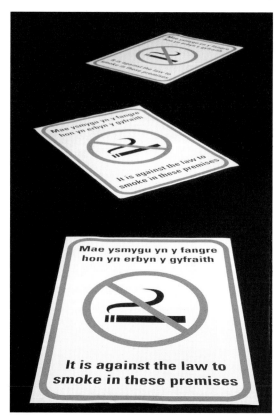

Bilingual no smoking signs 2007. (Science Museum, London)

jobs, apologies from the Health Secretary Patricia Hewitt and a judicial review of the system.

2006 **NHS Bowel Screening programme** is launched, offering home faecal occult blood testing, detecting an estimated 3,000 cancers each year

2007 **Smoking is banned** in restaurants, pubs and public places in England. A year after this, there is a significant decline in hospital admissions for heart attacks, asthma and lung infections.
Iphone launched

2008 **HPV (Human papilloma virus) vaccination programme** is launched to help prevent cervical cancer.
GP training – The RCGP publish a training curriculum for GPs and completion of the assessments for Membership of the Royal College of General Practitioners (MRCGP) becomes compulsory
The Darzi Review – High Quality Care for All is published led by Lord Ara Darzi, a colorectal surgeon and Minister. A year long review of the NHS is carried out, engaging 65,000 healthcare staff, patients and the public to discuss visions for the future of the NHS, and to examine barriers to delivering these visions.
Global financial crisis

2009 **The NHS Constitution** is published, setting out the rights and responsibilities of patients, staff and trust boards and the guiding principles which govern the service
The NHS Abdominal Aortic Aneurysm (AAA) screening programme is launched, aimed at detecting and treating large aneurysms early before they (often fatally) rupture. The screening programme invites men over the age of 65 to have an abdominal ultrasound scan to detect enlargement of the main blood vessel in the abdomen. This is not offered to women, as evidence suggests they are less likely to develop aneurysms than men, therefore screening can do more harm than good.
Swine flu epidemic
Barack Obama becomes the first African American president of the USA

My NHS Story

Hannah Ramsdale is a nurse on the neurosciences ward at the John Radcliffe Hospital in Oxford. She shares her experiences of the NHS.

'I qualified as an Adult Nurse (DipHE) in the summer of 2005. During my last few placements, in my third year of training, "Agenda for Change" was being implemented, to review and change nurses' pay structure and banding. I understood that upon qualifying I would become a Band 5 Staff Nurse and no longer a D Grade Staff Nurse. I can remember discussing it with my mentors and other nurses at the time and being incredulous about a question they were being asked in a survey about the changes: "Are you ever interrupted whilst trying to complete a task?" The exasperation, shock, irritation and laughter – as sometimes it's the only thing to do – I remember was from the nurses who would become my colleagues, and who knew, before I really did that the answer was yes. Persistently. Of course, we are.

'Every task, job, patient wash, dressing, drug round, handover, phone call, ward round, patient conversation, you are pulled and pushed in a variety of different directions: to a deteriorating patient, a colleague, urgent post-operative observations, doctor's instructions. I must also add that I became a nurse straight after completing my A levels. I have never known or worked in a corporate or business environment. This is all I know. I have now worked in the NHS for over a decade. I suspect most nurses may find my career path a bit backwards: most would have started out on the wards. However, once qualified I became a Band 5 Anaesthetic and Recovery nurse for Plastic and Neuro surgery, this lead me in less than a year to get a Staff Nurse position in Neuro Intensive Care (NICU), were I worked for four years. During this time, I travelled to Australia and worked as a Staff Nurse on a Medical Ward in Queensland. After leaving NICU in 2010 I held a brief community nurse role which then lead me back to the Neurosciences Ward, working with and caring for surgical patients, where I have worked for the last five years.

'I think in recent years, my experience of the NHS and especially in the ward I work, is that it is in constant motion. No sooner has a bed space has been cleaned and the bed made, another patient or even two, are already waiting for it. I'm not sure it is possible to move fast enough anymore. I find it extremely frustrating how much each department works separately to the next – in terms of respecting the enormity of each other's jobs and roles. We are all striving for the same thing. An absurd hierarchy of 'busy-ness' is maintained by all. The NHS isn't busy. It is overwhelmed. I'm not sure there is an accurate word to describe the environment, the system. People's lives are altered – and lost. Since I have been working in the NHS, I feel it is patient's expectations of it that are far too high. Expectations of what it is and what can be achieved. It has achieved such an incredible amount, and the public need that to be true for their mum, dad, auntie, uncle, brother and sister etc and when it isn't and either small things happen, or catastrophic events occur, blame must be placed and owned by someone. That is human nature. Though human nature is what is making every NHS Trust exist around the country in every staff member from our cleaning and clerical staff to Consultants and Directors and everyone in between.

'A keen interest of mine, that I've spent time highlighting on the ward is dignity and privacy. I found out about Dignity Champions in 2011, run by the National Dignity Council and have been holding Dignity Day events (held nationally on 1 February) on the ward each year. To find out from patients and relatives what we are doing well and those areas that need improvement. The smallest change can take the longest time to implement even with assistance of Senior ward management. It is always the little things that make a huge difference. I strive to do those small things as well as looking after my clinical caseload. Washing a lady's hair having waited a week after surgery. Cleaning a patient's glasses, helping a patient wash their hands before lunch. Brushing someone's teeth. Combing their hair. Putting on their favourite perfume/aftershave. It matters. I find my job a privilege. To care for someone at their most vulnerable is a privilege. The NHS horror stories that fill our news and conversations are real. Though I could give the same amount or more of wonder stories. Patients' lives that I'm unlikely to ever forget.

'What I think now though, is that I won't be a nurse till I retire. I am not quite ready to give up my registration just yet, but I honestly can't sustain the pressure of the environment, so very regrettably I can see that my skills need to be directed into a different area and role.'

2010s

The 2010s brought a series of NHS bad news stories – the Francis report, Budget deficits, patient dissatisfaction and emergency services in crisis. Increasing healthcare costs were driven by the ageing population, expensive new treatments and increased expectations. Ongoing austerity measures, pay freezes and imposed junior doctor contracts demoralized NHS staff, whose loyalty and goodwill notoriously kept the NHS afloat, leading to junior doctor strikes and an exodus of NHS staff overseas. Nonetheless, the public's affection for the NHS remained strong, and this was demonstrated and celebrated during the opening ceremony of the London 2012 Olympic Games. The passing of the Conservative government's 2012 Health and Social Care Act was one of the biggest reforms the NHS has ever seen, argued by some to mark the end of the NHS – not only by encouraging privatization and thus fragmentation, but by ending the duty of the health secretary to provide health services to the nation. The referendum on membership of the European union lead to a Brexit vote, and the UK Independence Party (UKIP) grew in strength. Seventy years on, the world is a different place to the post war era in which it was born, and the NHS is now way past retirement age, however, it is still standing. For how much longer, remains to be seen. The public of 1948, who stoically suffered through the Second World War are gone, and today we have a more atomised consumerist society, with a culture of instant gratification. Aneurin Bevan was famously asked how long the NHS would survive, and he replied 'As long as there are folk left with the faith to fight for it.'

2010   **Coalition government (Conservative/Liberal Democrats)**

2011   **Arab Spring**
        Greek Financial Crisis
        The NHS Constitution is published by the Department of Health to set out the guiding principles of the organization and be clear about the rights NHS patients and staff have. The NHS belongs to the people and the principals set by Bevan in 1948 remain core to the constitution, that it is free at the point of delivery, it meets the needs of everyone and is based on clinical need, not the ability to pay. All NHS bodies and private and third sector providers to the NHS are obliged by law to

take account of the constitution when making decisions. The constitution is renewed every ten years and any government that wishes to alter the principals and values of the NHS must first engage in a full and transparent debate with the public, patients and staff.

There are now seven key principals that guide the NHS:

- The NHS provides a comprehensive service to all
- Access to NHS services is based on clinical need, not an individual's ability to pay
- The NHS aspires to the highest standards of excellence and professionalism
- The NHS aspires to put patients at the heart of everything that it does
- The NHS works across organisational boundaries and in partnership with other organisations in the interest of patients, local communities and the wider population.
- The NHS is committed to providing best value for taxpayers' money and the most effective, fair and sustainable use of finite resources.
- The NHS is accountable to the public, communities and patients that it serves

UK riots following the death of Mark Duggan, a man shot dead by the police. Thousands of people rioted in London and other cities throughout the UK and the chaos this created led to looting, arson and 5 deaths. Racial tension and gang culture, combined with economic decline and unemployment have been debated as the cause for the breakdown in social morality seen during the riots.

2012   **The Health and Social Care Act 2012** – is passed in April 2013, bringing some of the most extensive reforms the NHS has ever seen. Since Bevan held the position in 1948, the Secretary of State for Health had been held responsible for providing a national health service, this Bill severed this duty and delegated it to CCGs (Clinical Commissioning Groups). PCTs (Primary Care Trusts) and SHAs (Strategic Health Authorities) were abolished and replaced by CCGs which were partly run by GPs but provided access for private providers. The Any Qualified Provider (AQP) scheme allowed private companies to compete for NHS funded work. It essentially legislated for reductions in government funded health services, while being unclear about who is ultimately responsible for people's health services, created new powers for charging and heralded a shift from tax funded healthcare to a one in which patients may have to pay.

Revalidation is implemented. All UK doctors are legally required to be revalidated every 5 years if they wish to retain their licence to practice. The process is based upon demonstrating up to date knowledge, by undertaking continuous professional development (CPD) and providing multisource feedback from patients and colleagues. The idea for revalidation was raised in the 1970s (The Merrison Report), but it was a series of high profile scandals (Shipman, Bristol heart scandal) that shaped the implementation of this process.

London 2012 Olympic Games – Danny Boyle pays tribute to the ethos of the NHS in his opening ceremony, celebrating free healthcare for all as a core value of British Society. The NHS was founded in 1948, but this was also the last time the Olympic Games had been held in London.

2013   **NHS England** forms to oversee the commissioning of NHS services in England and to set the priorities and direction of the NHS

Public Health England is formed as a result of the reforms. Prior to 2013, Public health operated through the PCTs (via the Department of Health's Health Protection Agency, and via the Strategic Health Authorities at a regional level). In April 2013, these responsibilities were returned to local authorities (where they had been up until the 1973 NHS reorganisations) and Public Health England was created as a distinct organization with operational autonomy from the government. The Department of Health restyled itself as a strategic director of both NHS England and Public Health England – meaning that the responsibilities to provide health care and public health services lies with these organization, rather than with the government themselves.

NHS Trust Development Authority is formed to oversee the management and governance of NHS Trusts

Healthwatch is created as a statutory accountability body, as the latest reorganization to involve patients and the public in the running of the NHS. 152 Healthwatch groups were established in each local authority area, and were allocated £43.5 million of the NHS budget to share ideas on how to improve health and social care services. Budgets have been cut each year, and their role has been criticized by the People's Inquiry into London's NHS, who believe the organization should be abolished

The Francis Inquiry Report is published, a public inquiry chaired by Robert Francis QC, examining the failings in care at the Mid-Staffordshire NHS Foundation trust between 2005-2009 – initiated due to its high mortality rates. Whole system failures are highlighted: Insufficient and inexperienced staff, insufficient training and a lack of beds and resources. Relatives spoke of family members being left in pain, unwashed and without access to food, water or the toilet. In 2006, the trust was tasked with saving £10million, and to achieve this, 150 staff were sacked and over 100 beds were taken away, resulting in a hospital unable to function, leading to situations where good people can do bad things. The 'Hard Truths' response to the inquiry announced that finances and targets would never again come before quality care and new safety schemes were proposed.

2014   **NHS ranked first** by the Commonwealth fund in a comparison of ten healthcare systems across the world (Australia, Canada, France, Germany, Netherlands, New Zealand, Norway, Sweden, Switzerland and the USA). The NHS comes top in terms of efficiency, safe and effective care, co-ordinated care, patient centred care and cost.

The NHS five year forward view is published, focusing on preventing patients getting ill and recognising the need for the NHS to adapt to our changing society. It sets out practical steps for the NHS to deliver a more joined up service based around new models of care, such as providing care traditionally delivered in hospital (like chemotherapy) in people's own homes and working in new ways – for example asking dementia specialists to conduct their clinics in GP surgeries, to improve access for those who need it.

Ebola outbreak in West Africa

Scotland votes to remain in the UK

Marriage (same sex couples) Act 2013 came into force and the first marriages take place in 2014

2015 **Conservative government**

Sustainability and Transformation Plans (STPs) are introduced in NHS planning guidance as part of the five year forward view to deal with the expected increase in demand for services coupled with the anticipated decrease in funding. They take a 'place based approach' focusing on NHS spending in named geographical areas across England, where leaders are asked to identify the key priorities for their local areas, and plan to improve efficiency of services by integrating with social care and local authority services, while delivering financial balance. NHS England describes STPs as collective discussion forums, which bring together organizations who have historically done their own thing. For example, the Lancashire and Cumbria STP brought together thirty-one different statutory bodies to discuss their area plans – nine CCGs, six NHS provider trusts, four local authorities and twelve district councils. Millions were spent engaging private management consultants in these plans.

Morecambe Bay Inquiry report published. Significant failures in care came to light at the maternity department at Furness General Hospital between 2004-2013, which may have contributed to the deaths of three mothers and sixteen babies. The report found poor working relationships between midwives, obstetricians and paediatricians and a 'them and us' attitude which hampered communication. Clinical competence among some staff fell below the expected levels, and a failure to perform adequate risk assessments, with an 'over-zealous' pursuit of natural childbirth by some midwives, led to unsafe care. Recommendations were to correct these problems, with an emphasis on reviewing serious incidents and learning from them. A national review of maternity provision in rural, isolated and difficult to recruit areas was advised.

2016   **Junior Doctors' strikes.** At a time when health spending is at its lowest since the Second World War, the government decides to push forward their plans for a 'seven day NHS' to extend the availability of non-emergency clinical services throughout the entire week – without providing the necessary planning, funding and staffing to do so. (It is worth highlighting here that emergency care is provided 24/7 already). The Morecambe Bay and Mid Staffs Scandals had demonstrated what happens when a service is poorly staffed, prompting proclamations that such poor care should rightly never happen again, but then the underlying issues of unsafe staffing and resources appear to be forgotten as the Health Secretary, Jeremey Hunt, makes the decision to impose the contracts for his vote winning 'seven day NHS', without coherently planning how he was going to deliver it. BMA negotiations break down, leading to strikes. The conflict is spun as a pay dispute, and the press label junior doctors as 'selfish, infantile, self-deluding idiots', igniting the fury of ordinarily placid junior doctors across the land, who are fearful of the implications of the contract. Being paid less is obviously

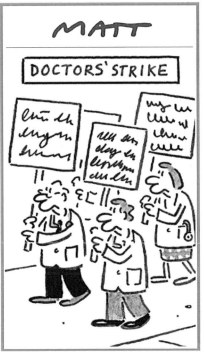

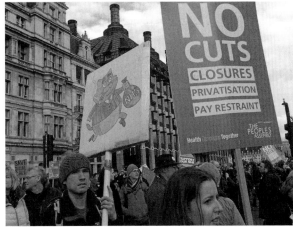

Save the NHS demonstration. (via Wikimedia Commons)

(© Telegraph Media Group Limited)

galling but stretching the already crumbling 5 day service over 7 days – without any extra doctors – would increase workforce strain, and ultimately reduce patient safety and quality of care.

The Cities and Local Government Devolution Bill is passed, allowing Secretaries of State to remove powers and duties from public bodies such as NHS trusts and commissioners, and transfer them to local councils or city authorities. This has raised concerns about just where accountability will lie in an increasingly devolved NHS.

NHS Improvement is launched to regulate all NHS providers as a merger of Monitor (which regulated NHS foundation trusts) and the Trust Development Authority (which regulated all other trusts)

Brexit – the UK votes to leave the European Union. The implications of this for the NHS remain to be seen but European migrants make up a significant proportion of the workforce and scrapping of regulations such as the EU working time directive will result in further staffing issues.

Donald Trump elected as president of the USA

2017   **Next steps on the NHS five year forward view** published by NHS England describing how its focus was evolving from STPs to Integrated Care Systems (ICSs) – also known as Accountable Care Organisations (ACOs) or Accountable Care Systems (ACSs) – which are population-based models of care inspired by US organisations, that integrate primary, secondary, community and other health services. The plan is for STPs to evolve into ACSs, in which commissioners, providers and local authorities join together to take collective responsibility for the health of their local area. Some areas may move towards ACOs, which are slightly different, in that commissioners in that area will hold a contract with a single organisation for the majority of health care provision

Staffing issues continue and the British Medical Association's annual representative meeting highlights significant gaps in doctor's rotas. Following a 2016 report from the Royal College of Physicians where 80 per cent per cent of doctors reported harmful and unsustainable levels of excessive stress at work, it was recognised that this was causing low morale and ever growing workloads.

RCEM Vision 2020 Following the worst four-hour performance in Emergency departments for fifteen years, The Royal College of Emergency Medicine makes a plan to fix the staffing, systems and support in Emergency departments. Since 2010/11, A&E attendances in England increased by 7.4 per cent per cent (equivalent to the workflow of ten medium-sized emergency departments), but the workforce and resources did not increase to meet this demand. More hospital beds and better integration of other services is called for to reduce pressure on A&E. Instead of spending £1.3million a day on locum staff (as is currently the case), the College also calls for increased consultant numbers and increased training posts.

The Lord Darzi Review of Health and Care interim report is published, a decade after his first report, to examine and reform the quality and funding of health and care services within the NHS. The full report is planned to be released on the NHS's seventieth birthday.

2018   **Hadiza Bawa-Garba** is struck off the GMC medical register in January 2018 after being found guilty of manslaughter on

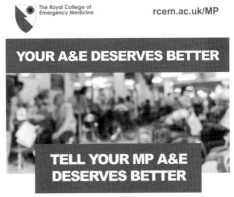

RCEM Vision 2020 Campaign. (Reproduced with permission from the Royal College of Emergency Medicine)

the grounds of gross negligence in 2015. In 2011, 6-year-old Jack Adcock was admitted to the Children's Assessment unit at the Leicester Royal Infirmary with diarrhoea, vomiting and difficulty in breathing. He had an underlying heart condition and Down's syndrome, which made the sepsis he was suffering with difficult to detect. A series of significant errors were identified in his care and he died later that evening after going into cardiac arrest. Paediatric trainee Dr Bawa-Garba was the ST4 Specialist registrar who treated him that day. She was alone, covering the Emergency Department and the Children's Assessment unit, with no senior consultant available on site. Rota gaps meant she was covering the work of two other doctors as well as her own, assessing multiple sick patients and, if this wasn't stressful enough, an IT failure in the hospital delayed any test results being available. She had also just recently returned from maternity leave. She was criticised for not specifically asking her consultant to review Jack – although she did share his clearly abnormal blood results with him during the evening handover meeting, and the consultant did not review on his own initiative. She was also criticised for not making it clear to Jack's mum that he should not receive his regular blood pressure mediation while he was unwell, and she deliberately did not prescribe this on Jack's drug chart. Tragically, Jack was given this medication, which, combined with the sepsis, led to circulatory shock and cardiac arrest. The case has raised debate about how medical errors are dealt with – particularly in this case, where system failures and the pressures of under-staffing all contributed to the death of a little boy, but the individual members of staff were singled out (Nurse Isabel Amaro was also struck off the Nursing Register for her involvement). Medics across the country spoke out at the verdict of this case, not to minimize or excuse the potentially avoidable death of a child – but recognising that the appalling working conditions Bawa-Garba was battling through that day allowed the negligence to happen. Recognising, with fear and vulnerability that the same conditions are occurring across the NHS every day, and that any doctor could be in the same position – #IAmHadiza.

Whistleblowing The case of Dr Chris Day is highlighted in view of the Bawa-Garba ruling. Junior doctor Chris Day raised concerns about under staffing in an Intensive Care Unit in London in 2013. Instead of tackling the patient safety issues raised, Health Education England (HEE) and the local NHS trust attempted to discredit Day and block his whistleblowing case being heard. GMC guidance clearly states that they will exercise statutory powers against doctors who do not take prompt action to deal with patient safety concerns, but when juniors do speak out there is no protection, and Day lost his career as a result. Whistleblowing doctors are marked as troublemakers in the management culture of the NHS, and the Francis Report identified this as a reason for the silence of many medical staff in Mid Staffs. Both Bawa-Garba and Day's cases highlight problems in the NHS culture in that you are 'damned if you do and damned if you don't'.

The Sugar Tax is introduced in an attempt to reduce sugar consumption and tackle obesity. Manufacturers of soft drinks are obliged to pay a levy on the high-sugar drinks they sell. Drinks with more than 8g of sugar per 100ml will face a tax rate of 24p per litre. The treasury expects to raise £240 million per year, which will be invested in breakfast clubs and school sports.

NHS70 Seventy years of the NHS is celebrated across the UK:

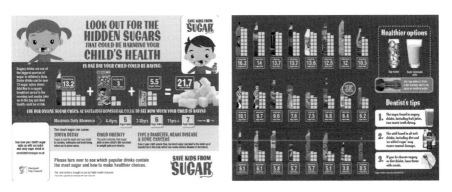

Sugar Cubes Campaign. (Used with permission from Public Health, Liverpool City Council)

My NHS Story

Dr Alison Gill is a Consultant in Respiratory medicine at York Teaching Hospital NHS Foundation Trust and shares her views on the NHS

'I joined the NHS in 2004, and have always found it both a pillar of UK life, and a perpetually-changing, ever more political machine. This perceived change may reflect the relative simplicity of the "house officer" life – mine was the last year before most hospitals transitioned to foundation programmes, and I was also one of the last to enjoy free hospital accommodation and the camaraderie this brought.

'House jobs were a fantastic year, with a busy but enjoyable job and amazing team spirit, combined with a good salary, my first experience of true financial independence, and a great social life. My medical career has always reinforced the idea that "if you want something doing, ask a busy person" as medics at university and since have always amazed me with their ability to have many other projects, hobbies and social events to balance their busy jobs.

'I can't think of a job I haven't enjoyed (though there are no shortage of less-than-enjoyable shifts) and I've been fortunate to use my medical training to work abroad in Africa and New Zealand, to travel as an expedition doctor, and to work in the medical centre at Glastonbury. While the politics and unclear future of the NHS make me try to ensure that prospective medical students understand the uncertainty, I usually undo this good work by telling them of my travels, and making them immediately press "send" on their University application forms.

'Over recent years, changes in medical politics have impacted particularly on juniors. The previously-revered medical registrar has become the first point of contact for routine tasks and even non-medical "emergencies" like a bird flying in through a ward window.... This excessive demand understandably deters many from higher medical training, resulting in ever-dwindling rotas and staffing shortages. At the same time, while working hour limits have improved safety and work-life balance, erosion of the traditional team has reduced continuity and the sense of belonging, while increasing bureaucracy has made training more of an administrative challenge. Political events such as the junior doctor contract dispute and strikes of 2016 have been hugely detrimental to junior morale, and an increasing sense of individual culpability is encouraging defensive practice rather than the balancing of risks and probabilities.

'This has escalated over recent years with a number of high-profile criminal prosecutions of doctors for gross negligence manslaughter in relation to medical error. An increasing public sense that human error is unacceptable in healthcare risks setting the patient safety agenda back by decades, as clinicians will be fearful of confessing to mistakes and near-misses. This is in direct contrast to both the NHS's professed blame-free culture, and to the duty of candour imposed since the Francis Report. It ignores the human factors which are so crucial to safe healthcare; these are recognised and embraced far more by the aviation industry, in which a genuine culture of honest error reporting has revolutionised safety records. Until the NHS truly embraces this safety agenda and moves away from blame in relation to error, such mistakes will continue and likely increase.

'Irrespective of this, I feel incredibly fortunate to work in such an interesting, varied and challenging profession, with some of the most dedicated people I can imagine. The NHS is, for all its faults, a fantastic institution of which the country is rightly proud. I believe passionately in the principle of healthcare free at the point of need and share Aneuryn Bevan's view that 'no society can legitimately call itself civilised if a sick person is denied medical aid because of lack of means'

Chapter 4

The Modern NHS

'I was to learn later in life that we tend to meet any new situation by re-organising, a wonderful method of creating the illusion of progress while producing inefficiency and demoralization'

Gaius Petronius – Roman Satirist 27-66AD

The NHS is a monolithic organisation, employing roughly 1.5 million people across the UK. The structure and administration of something so big is overwhelming. The sheer number of different organisations involved in the day to day running of the service is confusing even for those working within the service, especially given that these organisations have been renamed and rebranded each time a new government steps in, desperate to put their stamp on it. Seventy years of regular reforms with each successive government can be summed up in the quotation above.

For patients accessing the service, simply knowing where to go to seek help can be confusing. You stub your little toe and are worried it is broken – you go to your GP but can't get an appointment, the receptionist tells you that you will probably need an x-ray, which you can't get at the GP surgery. You go to hospital and wait four hours to be seen in A&E, only to be told by a grumpy triage nurse, that this isn't an emergency, you should have gone to the minor injuries unit. You go to the minor injuries unit, and are told, you can have an x-ray, but there is a bit of a wait, and after looking at the toe, the treatment will be the same with or without an x-ray. Your toe gets strapped, and you think that you could have done that yourself by visiting the pharmacy for some tape.

Even as a doctor working within the NHS, I became familiar with navigating how clinical services are intertwined, but understanding the management of the NHS, and how the government and various bodies interact was always a little hazy. The NHS is a national institution, and we all play a part in how it works – as patients, carers or employees. To improve a health service in crisis, it is essential for everyone using it to have an understanding of how it works, to be empowered to make it better.

NHS UK

The NHS was UK-wide when it was established in 1948, but decentralization in the late 1990s put control of all four countries health systems into the hands of each nation (England, Northern Ireland, Scotland and Wales), resulting in health service policies which are quite different. All of the UK has a tax funded service offering universal coverage, and the same core values. However, since devolution, reorganisations have occurred at different times, and policies have diverged. Prime examples of this can be seen by comparing England with Scotland, where free prescription drugs are provided, there is free personal social care for the over-65s and purchase of NHS funded care from private hospitals is discouraged.

The NHS in England is the largest and most market-oriented of the four, and what follows, focuses of the structure within the English system.

NHS England

Since the NHS is funded by taxes, it is inextricably linked to the government, and therefore politics. The Secretary of State for Health is head of the Department of Health – rebranded as the Department of Health and Social Care (DHSC) from January 2018. The government creates national policies and legislation and decides how much money

Table 4.1: The Department of Health and Social Care – Arm's length Bodies

NHS England	Leads the NHS in England by overseeing commissioning – the planning and buying of NHS services	https://www.england.nhs.uk
NHS Improvement	NHS Improvement oversees NHS trusts and independent providers to ensure high quality care which is, most importantly, financially sustainable. In April 2016, NHS Improvement was the rebranded name for the merging of 5 other organisations: -Monitor The regulator of NHS foundation trusts, which ensures they are financially sound and well governed -NHS Trust Development Authority (TDS) Formed in 2013 to be responsible for trusts unable to achieve foundation status -Patient Safety (including the National reporting and learning system (NRLS)) The National Patient Safety Agency (NPSA) was set up in 2001 to monitor patient safety incidents in a national database called the National Reporting and Learning System (NRLS). The NRLS allows similar incidents to be analysed to find common causes in an attempt to find solutions and avoid future incidents. NHS England took on the function of the NPSA in 2012, and NHS Improvement in 2016.	https://improvement.nhs.uk Monitor https://www.gov.uk/government/organisations/monitor NHS Trust Development Authority http://webarchive.nationalarchives.gov.uk/20161104155037/http://www.ntda.nhs.uk/ Patient Safety http://webarchive.nationalarchives.gov.uk/20160604124907/https://www.england.nhs.uk/patientsafety/ National reporting and learning system https://report.nrls.nhs.uk/nrlsreporting/Default.aspx

NHS Improvement	-Advancing Change Team Represented practical developmental learning programmes to help NHS staff and partner organisations to deliver change and improve services -Intensive Support Team Were external teams brought in to improve and support failing NHS organisations	Advancing change team http://webarchive.nationalarchives.gov.uk/20160506181459tf_/http://www.nhsiq.nhs.uk/capacity-capability/advancing-change.aspx Intensive support teams http://www.nhsimas.nhs.uk/ist/
Care Quality Commission	The CQC was previously known as the Healthcare Commission, and before that the Commission for Health Improvement and is essentially a regulatory body. The CQC monitors, inspects and regulates the standards of care provided by the NHS, local authorities, private companies and voluntary organisations, including independent hospitals, GP and dental surgeries, ambulance services and care homes.	http://www.cqc.org.uk
National Institute for Health and Care Excellence	Provides national guidance and advice to improve health and social care	https://www.nice.org.uk
Public Health England	Acts as the central organisation to lead public health initiatives such as health promotion, and immunization and screening programmes. Local health authorities took back responsibility for public health in 2013, and Public Health England provides overall leadership.	https://www.gov.uk/government/organisations/public-health-england
NHS Digital (previously known as Health and Social Care Information Centre)	The technological infrastructure of the NHS, uses data and technology to improve the NHS	http://content.digital.nhs.uk

(Continues)

115

Table 4.1 (*Continued*)

Health Education England	Delivers education and training for the entire NHS workforce. Made up of 6 advisory groups (to represent the interests of medical, dental, nursing, pharmacy, healthcare science and allied healthcare professionals) and 13 Local Education and Training Boards (LETB), who determine the local arrangements for the commissioning of education and training	https://www.hee.nhs.uk
Health Research Authority	Oversees health and social care research	https://www.hra.nhs.uk
NHS Blood and Transplant	Manages Blood donation and transplantation, researches new treatments and processes	http://www.nhsbt.nhs.uk
Medicines and Healthcare Products Regulatory Agency	Regulates medicines, medical devices and blood components in the UK	https://www.gov.uk/government/ organisations/medicines-and-healthcare-products-regulatory-agency
NHS Business Services Authority	Provision of central NHS services such as pensions schemes, payment of dentists and pharmacists, counter fraud, and determining the prices the NHS pays for consumables, including medication.	https://www.nhsbsa.nhs.uk NHS Pensions https://www.nhsbsa.nhs.uk/ nhs-pensions NHS help with costs https://www.nhsbsa. nhs.uk/nhs-help-health-costs NHS Prescription services https://www. nhsbsa.nhs.uk/nhs-prescription-services Information services https://www.nhsbsa.nhs. uk/information-services NHS penalty charges https://www.nhsbsa. nhs.uk/nhs-penalty-charges

Organisation	Description	Website
NHS Business Services Authority		Student services https://www.nhsbsa.nhs.uk/student-services NHS Dental services https://www.nhsbsa.nhs.uk/nhs-dental-services Total rewards statements https://www.nhsbsa.nhs.uk/total-reward-statements NHS Injury Benefits Scheme https://www.nhsbsa.nhs.uk/nhs-injury-benefits-scheme Supplier Management https://www.nhsbsa.nhs.uk/supplier-management Infected blood support scheme https://www.nhsbsa.nhs.uk/england-infected-blood-support-scheme NHS Protect https://www.nhsbsa.nhs.uk/nhs-protect-1
NHS Resolution (previously known as NHS Litigation Authority)	Manages claims against the NHS, resolves concerns about NHS professionals (including both clinical negligence claims and general claims such a occupational injuries). This is funded by annual premiums from trusts. The National Clinical Assessment Service (NCAS) is an operating division of NHS resolution, which helps to resolve concerns about the professional practice of doctors, dentists and pharmacists.	http://www.nhsla.com/Pages/Home.aspx
Human Fertilisation and Embryology Authority	Independent regulator of fertility treatment and research	https://www.hfea.gov.uk
Human Tissue Authority	Regulation of organizations involved with human tissue removal, storage, education and research	https://www.hfea.gov.uk
NHS Counter Fraud Authority	Investigation and prevention of fraud and economic crime within the NHS	https://cfa.nhs.uk

the NHS receives. The DHSC is supported by fifteen arm's length bodies (table 4.1) and a number of other agencies, external regulators and public bodies, which will be introduced below. Arm's length bodies are organisations that operate slightly apart from central government to conduct some of their business – meaning they are also easy to close down or re-organise if there are problems. They are also known as QANGOs (Quasi-Autonomous Non-Governmental bodies).

The bulk of the NHS piggybank goes to NHS England – an organization that was created in 2013 as a result of the Health and Social Care Act of 2012, in an attempt to distance the NHS from politics. NHS England effectively leads the NHS in England, setting the priorities and direction of the service. It was created as an independent special health authority to distance politicians from any operational responsibility. NHS England oversees the commissioning, planning and buying of NHS services, sharing out over £100 billion in funds to the 200 or so clinical commissioning groups (or CCGs) across the country. Some services, such as public health services, are commissioned directly by NHS England, but the bulk of commissioning is done by the CCGs.

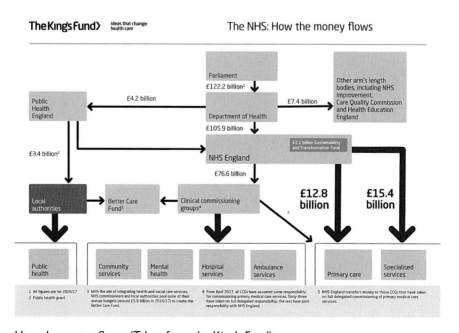

How the money flows. (Taken from the King's Fund)

NHS Commissioning

The current system for commissioning was implemented as a result of the Coalition government's Health and Social Care Act in 2012. The reforms created new organisations for the purchaser side, the provider side, and those to improve accountability for both (see table 4.2)

NHS England directly commissions specialized services, including renal dialysis, neonatal services and treatments for rare cancers. Primary care (including GPs, pharmacists, prison care, armed forces and dentists) and public health services are also directly commissioned. In 2016/17, NHS England had a commissioning budget of £105.9 billion. £28.2 billion was allocated for direct commissions, but the majority of this budget, £76.6 billion, wass allocated to local CCGs (see Fig 4.2).

Clinical Commissioning Groups, or CCGs, replaced Primary Care Trusts (PCTs) in April 2013, on the premise of moving the decision-making away from managers and back to clinicians. They have a statutory responsibility for commissioning most NHS services, such as emergency and urgent care, acute care, mental health and community services. They are increasingly involved in co-commissioning with NHS England some of the specialized services. Since 2015, NHS England has devolved responsibility for primary care to the CCGs – creating a structural conflict of interests, whereby the supposedly GP run CCGs commission themselves.

When first established in 2013, there were 211 CCGs, responsible for an average of a quarter of a million people each (although some

Table 4.2: Summary of the Health and Social Care Act 2012

Purchaser Side	Clinical Commissioning Groups The National Commissioning Board (Renamed NHS England in April 2013)
Provider side	Any Qualified Provider (AQP) Foundation Trusts
Regulators and accountability	The Care Quality Commission (CQC) and Healthwatch Monitor Health and Wellbeing Boards (HWB)

CCG populations range from 100,000 to 900,000). CCGs are made up of groups of local GP practices, which are led by an elected governing body (made up of GPs, nurses, secondary care clinicians and lay members). All GP practices have to be members of CCGs. This was a key principle of the 2013 reforms, which ministers used to defend the changes – as GPs were identified as the clinical group most aware of locals needs, priorities and services available, and most able to act as advocates for local communities. This sounds good in theory, but the reality of this is that overstretched GPs with a caseload of patients to care for, have little time or inclination to also take on the extra job of managing a budget of millions and planning services for their local areas. Most GPs opposed this, recognising they would be required to take the blame for rationing care to their own patients. In practice, CCGs are run by executive boards of managers, and GP involvement has been limited to small groups, rather than the GP community as a whole. Limited studies of CCGs have shown that the initial enthusiasm of some GP leaders to be involved had waned. A Lewisham GP wrote in the *Guardian* of the hours she spent acquiring the skills needed to lead commissioning in the local area, only to discover that the decision-making remained where it always had done – with the central managers – and the involvement of GPs was no more than window dressing for central planning geared towards the needs of the foundation trusts and private sector.

Local authorities are responsible for commissioning publicly funded social care services such as residential care and 'home help' services. About £15 billion was spent on adult social care in 2016/17. Until the late 1980's, long term care of the elderly was financed through the NHS and social security entitlements. This was removed by Margaret Thatcher's government and became the responsibility of local council social service departments, and people became subject to means tested charges. Today, most people in care homes pay for most of the costs of their own care. In 1979, 64 per cent per cent of residential and nursing home beds were provided by the NHS or local authorities -by 2012, only 6 per cent per cent. Domiciliary services such as home help schemes have also been privatised. In 1993, 95 per cent per cent of these services were provided directly by local authorities, and by 2012, it was just 11 per cent per cent.

Local authorities are also responsible for the commissioning of the public health services not covered by NHS England, including sexual health services, health visitors, school nursing and addiction services. The public health grant for local authorities for 2017/18 is ring fenced at £3.3billion (in 2017/16 it was £3.4billion). Health and Wellbeing Boards are formal committees that bring together local authorities and NHS representatives to carry out joint needs assessments with CCGs to develop joint strategies for their local populations.

CCGs and NHS England are supported by commissioning support units (CSUs) and from a range of private management consultants and voluntary sector organisations such as Capita, Optum and eMBED. These non-clinical support services are businesses which are themselves paid for with NHS money, to provide supporting back office services to the CCGs, such as IT, data management and HR support.

Any Qualified Provider (AQP)

To create a competitive market (especially for elective services), commissioners can procure 'any qualified provider', which has opened the door for non-NHS private companies to profit from the system. This was introduced as early as 2004, following the GP contract changes, which led to private providers taking over GP out of hours care. All providers must be accredited and licensed by the CQC, but any organisation with the required competencies can compete for NHS-funded work. This was one of the most contentious issues of the 2012 reforms, meaning that the internal market (where NHS providers competed for business from NHS primary care trusts) was no more. Instead, any organisation – private companies included – can compete for work. Common AQP services provided by private companies and third sector organisation (such as charities) include direct access MRI scanning, hearing aids and smoking cessation services. Private providers are notorious for cherry-picking less complex, more profitable patients and services, meaning that the NHS is left to deal with the more complex, costly cases that the private sector does not wish to provide.

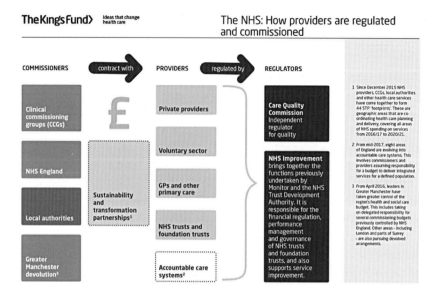

How providers are regulated and commissioned. (Taken from the King's fund)

Sustainability and Transformation Plans (STPS)

From 2015, some more acronyms were thrown into the mix. Sustainability and Transformation Partnerships or Plans (STPs) describe geographic areas of CCGs, local authorities and other local health care services that have united to plan and deliver healthcare. Their aim is to re-organise healthcare in a way that suits the local population. Money saving is a key driver of the plans, and service cuts are expected in favour of more integration of care. From 2017, Integrated Care Systems (ICSs) or Accountable Care Systems (ACSs) have evolved to basically do the same thing, but with a new name. The Plain English Campaign criticised the language of these plans saying they are 'vague enough to hide all manner of changes', while the BMA has questioned if NHS leaders actually have the budgets available to deliver the proposed projects.

NHS Finances

The money spent by the NHS is public money, raised from taxation. Each year, the government debates the annual budget, culminating in a vote to allocate money to the Department Health and Social Care, to spend on the health of the nation. The budget in 2016/17, was an estimated per cent£122.2 billion.

Since 1948, spending on the NHS has risen on average by 3.7 per cent each year. In 1950, the NHS spent an estimated £460 million. By 2020, it is likely to spend over 340 times as much – around £158.4 billion. Over this time period, increased costs and inflation would account for a lot of the spending, as well as increased medical innovations and more access to expensive technology and treatment. The aging population has also contributed, as well as inefficiencies in how it is spent

How much a country spends on healthcare, is ultimately a political and societal choice. Ken Loach says in the book *NHS SOS*, 'if the political will to sustain a publicly funded health service existed, a way would be found. If it were simply a matter of finance, there are solutions to hand' – such as gathering the billions of pounds of unpaid and uncollected taxes, along with the trillions that exist off shore to be used for the common good.

But equally, we have a responsibility as users of the service, to remember it is not a bottomless pit. In the UK, we are pretty ignorant about what healthcare costs. As an NHS GP, I have been asked to prescribe (often for wealthy patients, eligible for free prescriptions because of their age) toothpaste, sunscreen, vitamins and an entire grocery list of gluten free products. We as patients get grumpy if the GP asks us to go and pay for a 19p packet of paracetamol from a supermarket or pharmacy instead of getting it on prescription. Perhaps an awareness of the bigger picture would help. In 2016, the NHS spent more than £70 million giving paracetamol out on prescription. Once dispensing, consulting and administration fees are factored in, a prescription for 32 paracetamol can cost the NHS £34. NHS England launched a consultation at the end of 2017 to try to curb this spending, by asking that routine prescribing for self-limiting conditions stops. An estimated £136million could be saved by doing this, which could be re-invested in other areas of the NHS. Annually, the NHS spend £4.5 million on shampoos for dandruff (enough to fund 4,700 cataracts operations or 1,200 hip replacement operations) £7.5 million on indigestion and heartburn (enough to fund 300 community nurses) and £5.5 million on mouth ulcers (1,500 hip replacements). Is this a slippery slope in itself, that will lead to the poorest being denied the prescriptions they need? Personally, I think there needs to be a balance. In 1948, I very much doubt that patients were picking up their gluten free pizza bases and biscuits for free during a visit to see their GP – times have changed, and the system does need to adapt to change too. Does paying your taxes really entitle you to free toothpaste on prescription for your holiday to Myanmar (for which you have got first class seats)? – true story.

Perhaps this money could be spent instead on the woefully underfunded mental health services. More than 4,000 mental health beds have closed since 2010, coupled with a similar reduction in the number of psychiatric nurses. Access to these services is dire, as one service user recalls of her experience as an inpatient:

> 'I do feel in 2018 that mental health issues are talked about a lot more, which is as it should be. Life on a ward – you tend to walk around in circles trying to get cigarettes, tears, people screaming. We were all so unwell and had been removed from society. I was sectioned at various times over the past 40 years. Many locked wards that I've been on were tragically understaffed. It was an extremely unhealthy environment, with a shortage of compassion. If I became ill again today, I would find it very difficult to get a bed. I would need to travel more than 40 miles as so many psychiatric wards have been shut. On the upside, I have a decent enough mental health team, who I have a lot of faith in, but their job is difficult, with staff often off on long term sick.'

Regulation of professionals

Individual professionals within the NHS are regulated through bodies such as the General Medical Council (GMC), the Nursing and Midwifery Council, the Health Professions Council, the General Dental Council, the General Optical Council and the General Osteopathic council. The Royal Colleges and Specialist societies are membership organisations who have a range of responsibilities for ensuring standards of training in their particular areas, as well as improving service delivery.

The GMC

The GMC is the independent regulator of doctors in the UK. It is a registered charity whose purpose is to protect the public by ensuring good standards of medical education and practice. The GMC was formed under the Medical Act of 1858 in response to a census at the time, which suggested that a third of all doctors in England were unqualified. Today, it maintains a register of qualified doctors, including a specialist register of consultants and general practitioners – for which all doctors pay an 'annual retention fee' to maintain their name on the register. At the end of the seventies, this fee was £10 per annum, in 2018 it is £425, and failure to pay the fees can result in erasure from the register. It sets standards for medical education for medical schools and ensures doctors stay up to date through continuing professional development, and since 2012, through revalidation (see chapter 3). The Medical Act gives the GMC powers to take measures if questions are raised about a doctor's fitness to practise. Revalidation was introduced as a more proactive way of requiring doctors to demonstrate they are fit to practise and takes place every five years. Doctors who fail to engage with this will find themselves unable to practice, however the infrastructure of revalidation is almost entirely provided by the NHS – meaning that doctors without regular NHS employment, who may have previously plugged rota gaps, or provided NHS services in other ways, are unable to do so as easily as before.

Since the nineties, trust in the medical profession has declined following scandals such as Shipman, Bristol and Mid Staffs. However, the knee jerk reaction of stronger regulation to prevent this is not entirely evidence based, and the impact this has on professional motivation, and the health system as a whole is not insignificant. Doctors can be referred to the GMC by anyone, with no redress for groundless referral. Between 1992-2012, complaints to the GMC against doctor rose eight-fold. The number of public hearings increased five-fold, while the number of doctors erased from the medical register increased twelve-fold. Between 2003-2013, 96 doctors died while undergoing fitness to practice procedures (how many of these were suicide is unknown). In line with this inflation of claims, medical defence organisations (which all doctors are obliged to be members of) have increased their fees year on year to maintain cover for members subject to a GMC enquiry. As a full-time NHS salaried GP, I was paying £5000 annually. For locum and out of hours GP work however, I have been given quotes for over £9000 annually for cover. Have doctors become deviants? The GMC itself acknowledges that there is no evidence of a decline in standards of medical practice to justify their increased activity. Furthermore, there is no published evidence, that GMC fitness to practise processes improve the quality of medical care given to patients. There is evidence however, that a complaint culture results in the practice of defensive medicine. Doctors dealing with claims often give up clinical practice, or report feeling more distant from their patients. The question must therefore be asked – is the GMC fit to practice, when its own activity seems to take no regard of its impact on both doctors and patients?

NHS Staff

The NHS is haemorrhaging staff. As the workload and conditions become worse, more and more undervalued staff opt to throw in the towel to go elsewhere. Figures from OECD show that the UK has fewer doctors per head than most of Europe – 2.8 doctors per 1000 people, which is below the OCED average of 3.4. Like the Eurovision results, we perform poorly compared to most of our neighbours such as Greece who has the most at 6.1, but Portugal (4.6), France (3.3), Estonia (3.4) and Latvia (3.2) all fare better than us. The NHS is desperately short of nurses, and figures from early 2018 show that across England, only 1 in 7 of all empty nursing posts were filled. GPs too, face a recruitment crisis, and despite a government pledge to increase GP numbers by 5000 by 2020, the number of full time equivalent GPs fell by 0.3 per cent per cent in 2016. GP workload has grown in recent years, not only in volume, but in complexity, and experienced GPs are seeking early retirement, whilst newly qualified GPs opt for portfolio careers, combining clinical work with teaching, research, or anything other than the daily slog of full time GP work. Given the long training times for clinical professionals, there are concerns over whether the NHS can recruit and retain enough staff to meet the growing demands on the service.

Those staff that remain are undervalued. Junior doctors in particular, are uniquely exploited by management, who are aware that they are unlikely to complain and risk their future employment at a trust. Junior doctors have often been doctors for many years, but until they become a consultant, training programmes mandate them to rotate to different hospitals every 3-12 months – which in itself can be isolating and demoralising, working shifts with different colleagues each day, with no time to build relationships before moving on again. Trainees are routinely posted to work in hospitals miles away from their homes – often only getting their rotas a few days prior to a changeover. Rota gaps are expected to be covered. Some surgical trainees are required to work a full day and then be on call overnight – sometimes from home. Some hospitals have mandated these doctors to remain on the hospital site overnight if their homes are too far away – and in these cases, on call rooms are provided by the hospital. One surgical registrar spoke of being sent a bill for the use of this room and threatened with debt collectors if he did not pay. Worried about his career, he paid, for a room he was too busy to use, a room that would be sitting empty anyway, and a room he didn't want in the first place.

My NHS Story

Dr Neil Barnard is a South African medical graduate who completed his intensive care and emergency medicine training within the NHS. He recently moved his family over to New Zealand to live and work, and he shares his reasons why.

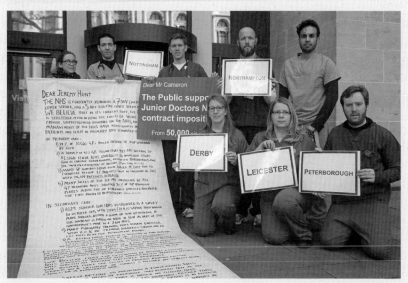

Midlands Junior Doctors outside the Department of Health (Neil Barnard second from right, back row) (Photo taken by Matt Saywell - copyright of the British Medical Association)

'I came to work in the NHS initially via the UK private system, followed by a stint as a ship's physician in the Caribbean, further experience in South Africa, and training in Australia before, having met my English wife, begrudgingly returning to England to live and work there.

'I am not wedded to the NHS because of some sort of national pride, political ideology or religious fervour. I was, in fact, a reluctant NHS worker when I first arrived to take up an emergency medicine post in Coventry. I was under no illusions when I left Australia to go to the UK. I knew that my lifestyle would be much worse, my pay would be no better and the weather would be abysmal. Yet, despite this, I was excited to have the opportunity to work in a system which valued doctors, was consistently rated as one of the most efficient in the world, put patients before profit and would provide excellent, world class training.

'I arrived in the August of 2010, incidentally, three months after the Conservative party became the major part of a coalition government.

'My first professional experience of the NHS was very rewarding, I worked in a motivated, extremely busy emergency department which had been newly built in the last five years. The workload, though intense was neither demoralising nor unmanageable. I worked with a group of colleagues and senior clinicians who were supportive of each other and felt rewarded in the work they did. Most importantly, the nursing staff were mostly, staff who had been in the department for a number of years and formed a stable and caring base upon which the department was built.

'So, what happened between then and August 2017 when, in the space of just seven years, despite having lived in the UK, bought a house, and had children who were starting to settle in school, I discussed matters with my wife and took the big decision to relocate our family to New Zealand? New Zealand, where neither of us had ever been; where we had neither friends nor family and where it would take either of us a day and a half of flying to get home if we needed to.

'In short, the NHS had begun a slow and apparently unchecked spiral towards an underfunded, under-resourced service. A decline which allowed pay for NHS workers to be frozen for seven years resulting in a real term cut for some staff of 30 per cent per cent. A decline which allowed the NHS budget, despite claims to the contrary, to be cut in real terms, when demands for acute services had never been higher yet staff numbers in terms of staff per attendance ratio had never been lower.

'In an unprecedented event in 2016, junior doctors, a largely homogenous group of uncomplaining, professional people who happily stayed extra hours and sacrificed their own time and effort for the good of their patients, went on strike – not over pay but in protest against the way the NHS has been eroded. The way staff have been unsupported and conditions have deteriorated to a point where patient safety has been compromised as a result of doctors not being able to provide the level of care they want to for their patients.

'In the last two years, we have heard countless news stories about nurses using food banks to survive to the end of the month and nurses being balloted about potential strike action. In my own department, nursing turnover was so high that having spent 18 months doing subspecialty training in a different department, I returned to find that I no longer knew most of the nurses working there. Burnout, exhaustion and record numbers of staff retirements and absence due to sickness have all lead to a massive reliance on locum staff who neither know or care for the departments as much as those staff who had previously committed to the team.

'By the time, I had come to the end of my training in the UK, despite having a dual qualification in intensive care and emergency medicine which afforded me the pick of jobs anywhere in the country, I could not face working feeling as if my back were constantly against the wall. I could not face feeling as if we were shuffling the deck chairs on the *Titanic* while our politicians instructed the band to play on, oblivious of the looming crisis.

'It turns out, I left at the right time. I am still a member of the local trainee group at my former trust. It is heart breaking this year to hear stories of patients piled up in corridors, of record ambulance waits, of record waiting times to be seen in the department and hearing the stories of mental, physical and emotional exhaustion from my colleagues who are some of the hardest working people I've had the privilege to work with. It galls more when on the BBC news, the politicians of the day, can only talk about how well they were prepared for the winter. It is clear that they were never prepared and their empty thanks for the hard work being put in by NHS workers across the spectrum of care feel like empty platitudes.

'Perhaps I should not have been surprised when I arrived in New Zealand and found that 60 per cent per cent of the junior medical staff in my new department were UK graduates. I should also not have been surprised that almost all of them have no plans to return to the country of their birth. When one considers the differences in conditions, it really isn't surprising at all.

'We work in a department where staff numbers are adequate and necessary resources are provided. Nursing numbers follow recommendations applied by the Australasian College of Emergency Medicine. Training is an integral part of the system and consultant staff have the time to teach while junior staff have the time to be taught.

'A work/life balance is recognised as a vital part of staff happiness and productivity such that sickness rates are much lower and staff are motivated and keen to come to work. The trust recognises the work that we do and values us sufficiently to pay for professional indemnity, professional registration and ongoing clinical development.

'The work is certainly not of a lesser standard or complexity. I am challenged daily but, importantly, I feel supported by my colleagues, the hospital and the Health System as a whole. It appears that the system that was largely based on NHS principles and has always looked up to the NHS has now got much to teach the NHS in return.

'I have no desire to return to the NHS unless a fundamental commitment is made which will help turn things around. Until then, I can look forward to the ongoing steady stream of former colleagues sending me their CVs and asking about vacancies.

'Shame. The once proudest achievement of post war Britain is no more. How the mighty have been allowed to fall.'

Please let us work

Amidst our NHS workforce crisis, where GP leaders and politicians proclaim that urgent measures should be taken to invest in recruitment to boost GP numbers, there exists a cohort of qualified GPs who are desperate to return to the UK to work as GPs but are being strangled by red tape.

Any doctor wishing to work as an independent, unsupervised GP in the UK, is required to:

1 be on the GMC GP Register (which means completing 5-6 years of medical school, and working at least 5 years as a doctor)
2 Hold a GMC licence to practise
3 Be on the National Performers' list

There are three performers' lists operated by NHS England (for medical, dental and ophthalmic performers) that exist to provide another layer of reassurance for the public that professionals practising in the NHS are suitably qualified, with up to date training, can speak English and have passed relevant checks (such as with the Disclosure and Barring Service [DBS]). Performers' lists came into operation in April 2004 (a result of the Health and Social Care Act [Community Health and Standards] 2003), as a reaction to cases of dodgy doctors in the NHS (notably, Shipman), to create a formal process to ensure quality.

This means that experienced GPs who did not train in the UK, and doctors who have been out of UK general practise for two years, must jump through a series of expensive and time consuming hoops before they can join or re-join the NHS workforce. Overseas doctors must first obtain the Certificate of Eligibility for GP Registration (CEGPR) – a process that often takes up to twelve months, collecting documents and providing evidence. Instead of reviewing each doctor on a case by case basis, and considering their experience and merits, both overseas doctors and returning UK doctors then all have to go through the GP Induction and Refresher Scheme (I&R Scheme) – another process which can take another twelve months to navigate. Having these safeguards is understandable, to ensure GPs working in the UK are familiar with the NHS and are up to date after long periods out of practice – but blindly subjecting all returning GPs to the same process if they do have the experience and qualifications is a waste of valuable time and resources which could be better spent providing a service to the public and reducing GP waiting times. To add insult to injury, this process costs money. To obtain the CEGPR, one doctor calculated expenses of over £2,000 for the whole process, and for the I&R scheme, almost £5,000 – not including the loss of income for the entire time they were not working. Many GPs opt to remain overseas, or throw in the towel completely, and pursue alternate careers, rather than put themselves through this process. Is it any wonder we have no GPs, if coming back to work in the UK is this much hassle?

GP I&R Scheme case study

Dr Irina Bardsley qualified as a UK GP in 2013, after completing a formal three year speciality training programme in the North of England as a GP Registrar. She co-authored a book to help fellow trainees pass one of the exams required to become a GP, and then went to work as a GP in New Zealand for three years with her husband.

During her three year period away from UK general practice, she worked continuously as a general practitioner in New Zealand in what the GMC and Medical Council of New Zealand (MCNZ-NZ's GMC equivalent) describe as a 'comparable healthcare system'. She was required – as part of the MCNZ's registration requirements – to be enrolled in a portfolio system almost identical to those used in the UK to revalidate and appraise doctors. This involved completing a minimum set of annual CPD activities, audits, multi-source feedback, and patient feedback cycles. She maintained her registration with the GMC, but, on the advice of her UK appraisal lead, resigned from the performers list.

She returned to the UK for family reasons in 2017, with two job offers before she had even booked her flights home. She returned to the city in which she had trained, where practices had struggled to recruit GPs for years. She was known to the staff and patients she would be working for. Her local performers' list invited her to a meeting to review her documents and welcomed her with open arms, thrilled that a UK-trained GP had returned to the country. The day before she was due to start working at the surgery, the performers list contacted her again to say sorry ... but she had been out of the UK for too long and could not work until she had completed the I&R scheme. The performers' list staff actually had no idea what was required and were unable to provide any guidance. This was the beginning of a lengthy process of paperwork, assessments, and mindless red tape which meant she was unable to work as a GP for more than six months.

The I&R scheme decided that anyone who had not served a minimum of two years working as a GP *prior* to moving overseas, does not qualify for the 'Portfolio Route' whereby Irina's evidence could have been reviewed to allow her to continue working in the same country that she trained and qualified in. Instead of looking at each individual doctor's circumstances, on a case-by-case nature, to allow those that have an exceptional level of evidence to simply continue to practice medicine, the scheme stops good doctors from working.

For Irina, what came next, was a series of demoralizing assessments, a simulated surgery exam – similar to the exam she had written a book about – and then supervised placements. Firstly came clinical multiple choice questions, aimed at more junior doctors working in a hospital setting 'imagine you are an SHO in A&E or an F2 on the ward...' and questions about procedures that would never be carried out in primary care (consenting patients for specialist surgical procedures, or thrombolysing a Pulmonary embolism). For an exam that is supposed to be geared up for GPs that are fully qualified and practicing, it is questionable if it is fit for purpose. Following this was a Situational Judgment test, where candidates are asked to rank their actions in order of appropriateness. Actual questions include: 'a patient's dog has passed away, would you: advise her to get a dog from the shelter; give her one of your puppies that your own dog recently had; ask her to seek support from a friend...' or 'A nurse asks you to help move furniture from one room to another while you are doing your surgery, please rank in order...'

How is this a superior method of assessing a GP's competence than reviewing actual evidence supplied from a medical council from another country with a similar healthcare system? The scheme is arguably a detriment to a doctor's clinical practice, in that they are removed from day to day clinical contact with patients for several months, to spend time relearning questions to pass an exam.

Working abroad arguably makes people better GPs, not worse. In some countries, it is actually encouraged to spend time working abroad before being fully signed off in a speciality. There is no other speciality in the UK that requires additional assessments to get back to work (including independently practicing medical consultants) – Irina's husband, for example was able to simply pick up where he left off three years earlier in hospital medicine, without the rigorous scrutiny and loss of earnings imposed on GP returners.

The I&R scheme is damaging the morale of previously enthusiastic GPs, keen to bring their overseas experiences back to the NHS, but find they are unable to work due to numerous (and arguably unnecessary) assessments. Even GP registrars in training are allowed to work independently (under the supervision of an allocated GP) – so why is it so difficult for fully qualified GPs to return to practice, particularly those who haven't even had any time out? Why can't the scheme allow GP returners to arrange their own jobs (effectively being screened by an individual GP practice) and simply complete a minimum period of supervision without unnecessary exams that are forcing us to take time out of practice, placing undue and unfair strain on good GPs from a financial, practical, and even mental-health perspective?

Private Healthcare and the USA

The Commonwealth Fund reported in 2014 that the NHS was rated top on quality of care and access to care, while the US, where the private sector provides healthcare, was most expensive and the worst performing. The US assigns 18 per cent per cent of its economy to health spending – double that of the UK, but is near the bottom in measures of health and life expectancy compared with sixteen other economically wealthy countries.

Healthcare costs in the States are notoriously steep. In many hospitals, doctors' pay depends upon the procedures their patients have – meaning that financial incentives can impact on the care given. As George Bernard Shaw wrote at the turn of the twentieth century, giving people a financial interest in cutting your leg off can have some pretty obvious drawbacks. A colleague in the States spoke of a medical bill amounting to $86,000 when his father passed away at home, and healthcare professionals did little more than declare him dead. His family called 911 when his father collapsed with a cardiac arrest. The paramedics charged a fee for every mile it took them to reach his home in the ambulance, in addition to the fee charged to dial 911 in the first place. They charged for the act of unloading their equipment from the ambulance, a fee to enter the house, another charge for starting CPR, for picking him up from the floor to a stretcher, more costs to move him to the ambulance, charges to open their bag and for every medication and disposable item used during their visit – even down to the gloves worn by the paramedics and the piece of paper used to cover the stretcher his father lay on. The fee to declare him dead alone was $7,000.

A day in hospital in the US costs over ten times more than in other countries and patients get more tests and more interventions – driven by profit and fear of litigation, rather than from practising good medicine. Instead of sharing risk and uncertainty, patients are over-investigated and over-treated. Popular doctors will attract more customers, and popular doctors will often be the ones that give customers what they want. Antibiotics for their runny nose that started this morning; IV opioid analgesia for the sprained ankle ... I work as both an NHS GP and as a cruise ship doctor for an American company. On cruise ships, guests pay for the medical services they receive. They also fill out guest satisfaction surveys at the end of their vacation where they rate the cruise. The fact they ended up in the medical facility already means they probably didn't enjoy their vacation due to being unwell, and then when we don't provide a 'Z-pack' (antibiotics) or Vicodin (narcotic) on request, or even worse if we isolate them for public health reasons to prevent an outbreak – we will hear about it in the survey. Similar 'rate my doctor' surveys exist in the US, and it is easy to see how as a doctor, it is easier to give a patient what they want to keep them happy (boosting ratings and profits) rather than having a difficult conversation – but this is not good medicine. To take the example of antibiotic prescribing – most of the American guests I see with a cold on the ship come to see me expecting to be able to pay for antibiotics as they do back home (antibiotics are not needed for a self-limiting illness – Public Health England have developed antibiotic guardian resources if you want to read more http://antibioticguardian. com/). It would be much easier for me to smile and hand them over to this paying customer, than to take the time to explain the reasons why they are not needed or going to make them feel better – it risks confrontation and the likelihood of being blamed on the satisfaction survey for the fact they coughed for the entire vacation. Similar dilemmas arise in the NHS, and GPs have been threatened with being reported to the GMC for refusing to prescribe antibiotics for a cold.

At the opposite end of the private medicine spectrum, are the situations on board, where we are compelled to discuss the cost of treatment with patients to ensure they are happy to pay the fees. The medication used to bust the clot causing a heart attack costs $7,000. I have been in a situation where the patient is in a critical condition and I have been stopped by the nurse to go and check with the person paying the bill that they are happy for us to administer this potentially life-saving treatment, at a cost of $7,000. In the NHS we don't have to worry about these issues ...yet.

A study in the NEJM in 1997, concluded that almost 100,000 people died in the United States each year because of a lack of medical care, due to being unable to pay for medical insurance. Insurers limit their risks by selecting out the poor, the elderly, those with mental health problems, homeless people and migrants. Even among those who are insured, many fall ill, only to find they have inadequate coverage, and have to live with the fear of healthcare bills.

NHS Privatisation

Private companies have been part of the NHS for years. It started in the eighties with support services such as portering, catering, cleaning and IT being provided by private companies. Following the 2004 GP APMS contract changes, which allowed non-NHS providers to provide primary care services, private companies such as Virgin started to take over GP out of hours services. The following year, Independent sector treatment centres were introduced. The scale of private companies' involvement in the NHS accelerated following the 2012 Health and social Care Act, to involve GP surgeries, urgent care and minor injuries units, community services, maternity care, ambulances, diagnostic imaging, prison care and even whole hospitals and A&E departments. Private consultancy firms are increasingly being used in health planning – in the form of commissioning support units and accountable care organisations. In 2016/17, almost 70 per cent of the 386 clinical contracts put out to tender went to the private sector (worth £3.1 billion), with Care UK and Virgin Care holding the largest share of these. This may not be obvious to patients using the service, since all these private providers are encouraged by the Department of health's branding team to use the NHS logo, without using their own.

Is this a problem? The priority of private companies is to provide a profit for the shareholders, meaning when it comes to healthcare, they are unlikely to get involved with services that are expensive to deliver. While the UK public sector continues to be cut back, the services deprived of the resources, such as emergency care, care for the elderly and the chronically sick, are the areas that private providers avoid at all costs, since they are complex, risky and unprofitable. Private hospitals in the UK, on the whole, are set up to treat elective cases – typically healthy patients undergoing routine, less risky procedures. UK private hospitals are not required to teach or train their staff. The headlines that undermine the NHS often put the alternative option of private care on a pedestal, as if poor care couldn't possibly happen there. I recall as a junior doctor, working in an NHS hospital, having private patients transferred to the care of the NHS as soon as they became too unwell to handle. Even as a GP, I was visiting a patient having chest pain in a rural area who asked me as we waited for the ambulance if they should use their insurance to go to a private hospital for treatment, and my answer was no – the local private hospitals are fine for your routine knee replacement, but they are not where you want to be if you are acutely unwell with a likely heart attack. It is not possible to deliver universal healthcare through a market system, as it makes no money. To quote author Simon Sinek: "When people are financially invested, they want a return. When people are emotionally invested, they want to contribute". This is why a publicly funded and owned NHS is seen as among the fairest and most efficient in the world – when funded properly.

Medicine and the Media

The media shoulder a huge responsibility when it comes to informing the public about the NHS and about healthcare in general. How information is reported has an influence on people's perceptions – as was demonstrated during the MMR vaccine scare (where media coverage did not align with the weight of scientific evidence, leading to unvaccinated children and re-emergence of measles). Sadly, the vast majority of mainstream media reporting on the NHS is scaremongering propaganda, peddled by the politicians. My grandmother, a staunchly working class labour voter from Newcastle, now in her 90s, like many from her generation, would never think to question what the newspapers were telling her. If it wasn't true, then it wouldn't be on the news would it?

A study at Cardiff university in 2007 found that journalists were producing more content than they were 20 years before, but only 12 per cent of stories were being properly checked. Complexity, details and accuracy are compromised, and the speed at which erroneous or unfair allegations can be published has far reaching implications. Journalists work to deadlines, and it is easier to regurgitate a government press release, than to wade through the rhetoric to report the facts. Furthermore, explaining the complexity of the problems in the NHS, is going to take more than the 500 words allocated to most reporters.

The NHS winter crisis, which has extended into a year-round problem, is a result of the government imposing years of austerity measures. Insufficient hospital beds and a lack of social care to discharge the patients in said beds, means the new patients attending A&E are stuck on trolleys for hours. The money that should have been spent on these services, was instead wasted on the NHS reorganisations designed to privatise the NHS. The Department of Health controls the health news agenda, and their press releases blame the inappropriate attendees, the GPs and the hospital managers and their solution is for the public to realise we need to start to pay for our care – scare tactics designed by the government to push forward their agenda of privitisation.

Journalists love human interest stories, and when it comes to the NHS there is an endless supply. Doctor bashing in particular, has become a national sport, reaching a peak during the recent junior doctor strikes. In a post-Shipman world, allegations against doctors make good copy, and are justified in the public interest. Poor care should rightly be flagged and rectified, but there are always several sides to a story. Patients who sell their stories are not bound by any codes of confidentiality, whereas healthcare professionals certainly are, meaning correcting inaccuracies in the story may risk breaching confidentiality, and the true events of any scandal may not be what make the headlines.

Serial killing doctors sell papers, but even the fairly boring ones can provide a good story if the facts are twisted around sufficiently. In January 2018, hundreds of senior doctors took a break from the NHS's worst winter emergency to enjoy a taxpayer subsidised conference at a luxury alpine ski resort. The *Mail on Sunday* told us about overflowing A&E departments, and patient's having their operations cancelled, while the doctors who should be treating them had waltzed off to France to knock back champagne and slalom down the slopes. The purpose of the story was to incite indignation, to undermine doctors, to sow the seeds of discontent with the public, so that when doctors vocalise their concerns about the NHS, the public can be reminded that doctors are in it for themselves. While I would hazard a guess (since I have not interviewed or researched the facts of this particular story, but recognise the situation from my own experience of working in hospitals) that the reality of the story would be more along the lines of: doctor decides a year in advance to attain their compulsory educational requirements by attending a medical conference based at a ski resort, to combine the time they are able to claw away from work with a bit of a holiday alongside some education. Study leave was denied by the employers, so a week of annual leave is used, by swapping their rota with three others and doing a week of nights to compensate. The cost of the conference cannot be covered because they have already used up their study budget for the year, and spent another few grand on top of that undergoing further training and exams.... Not such a snappy headline grabber.

The GMC has investigated doctors based on nothing more than a media report. An NHS colleague spent some time working for an online pharmacy, which was regulated by the CQC, with safeguards in place for prescribing over the internet. A journalist, in search of a story, placed a fraudulent request to the site, requesting the weight loss pill orlistat. They filled out the online questionnaire which checks medical history, height, weight, contraindications to the medication and asks patients to confirm they are telling the truth. The journalist lied about their weight and height, saying they were obese when they had a normal BMI. The pill was provided, a scathing article was published, and the doctor prescribing the pill was referred to the GMC for further investigation. Where is the accountability for the damage caused by irresponsible reporting?

My NHS Story

Carol Trow is a full time author and editor who previously worked for the NHS and in the private sector until 2000 as a biomedical scientist. She shares her experiences as a user of the service, in a blog post that was originally written for the *Huffington Post* – 'No one wants to hear the NHS good news!'

'Five weeks ago, the unthinkable happened, right there, on the sofa; my previously healthy husband had a heart attack. I dialled 999 and dragged him off the sofa in one movement and within seconds was performing CPR. And screaming at him. Then the paramedics arrived and I heard the dreaded word – "Clear!" – and then silence; I have to admit, for a while there, it's a bit of a blur.

'Then suddenly, he was away from me, in an ambulance and the chaos that is A&E awaited. But ... and here comes the bit that news media doesn't want to hear … the staff were all fabulous, the care he got was exemplary. There were no trollies in the corridors, no dirt, no mess, no waiting. Just a team all gathered round him, adding tubes and leads; arranging a bed in a nearby centre of excellence; sorting an Air Ambulance. Reception staff were patient, while dealing with dingbat members of the public abusing them because my husband had "jumped the queue".

I was hugged, consoled, told the truth – he might not make it, but if he didn't, it wasn't going to be because he wasn't fighting or that I had done anything wrong in the CPR. He was packed up like a Christmas parcel and loaded onto the helicopter on the way to QAH, in Cosham.

'And then, the waiting. And the discovery that, pressured and beleaguered though it is, the NHS can really pull out all the stops, if you do the same. My husband, chilled to 36 degrees, intubated, sedated, with a balloon pump to keep his heart going, perhaps didn't look as if he was bringing much to the table, but my word, that man's a fighter. My son and his wife and baby son were with us on the long trip back to normal. And all the time, the nurses and doctors were by our side, caring, professional and I don't hesitate to say loving. We got attached to "our" first nurse, Ben, who quietly changed his next shift so he would be there next day as well. There was Liz, Edwin, Christian, Francisco, Claire, May, Edgar, Peter, David … the list is endless of people who know their jobs inside out and how to go the extra mile.

'We were warned that we might not get "him" back, except in body as he may have had oxygen deprivation in the first minutes after the attack. But, he *is* back. He doesn't remember the actual event or the few days before it and his memory of his hospital stay is sketchy to absent, but everything else is fine; fine because someone in that A&E saw that he could make it; because the air ambulance and two centres of excellence were there; that the nurses, doctors, physios, all gave their time and love without condition. And because he wasn't ready to go – but spirit alone is nothing without the NHS.

'So – NHS knockers; Stop It! Time wasters – go to your pharmacy if you feel a bit under the weather. Read what it says on the sign; "Accident and Emergency". It doesn't say "Feeling a bit iffy and want some medicine". Cussers and swearers – keep it to yourself.

Being writers, we thought, hey – let's get to the media, tell them how fabulous everyone has been. We're not uber-famous, but eighty books is no small feat, he's been on telly as well, so we thought that the local media at least would print this feel-good story. But no. We didn't even get a phone call, an email in reply. It turns out that good news is no news.

'If we have learned anything, it is this. Don't listen to all the news about lines of grandmas left to languish on trollies in corridors. Don't listen to the stories about filth and "third world care". Listen to the *real* news that isn't news, that the NHS is alive and well – if a little underfunded. And get out there, do what you can to help the funding. We write, so that's what we're going to do. Our daughter-in-law is doing a run. Our son is putting on an all-day music fund raiser. Everyone can do something to help. But most of all, love and cherish our NHS – like the NHS, 70 years old this year and feeling her age, loves and cherishes us.

The Future

Is the NHS going to make it to its 80th birthday celebrations? The NHS is a set of principles about the way we value healthcare. It borders on being a national religion, and still retains huge public support. We need the NHS. Politicians with their private health insurance perhaps don't, but the majority of people in this country rely on the service, and to ensure it endures and functions, we all need to make what we have work better. As Margaret McCartney advocates in her book the state of medicine – we need less short term political policy making when it comes to the NHS, and more decisions made based on evidence and expertise.

It is clear there is an abundance of problems with the NHS, but I do feel strongly that privatising it will not make the service better. To declare my conflicts of interest, I have experience of both systems – I trained in the NHS and undertake locum GP shifts at an NHS practice in London to maintain my place on the performers' list. My main job at present, is on cruise ships – which is a mix of private healthcare (guests pay) and free healthcare (crew don't). I have dabbled in private medicine, I tried working as a GP on Harley Street but it wasn't for me, and I have recently started working for a private company offering telemedicine services.

To save the NHS, we need to be better informed about what is going on. Many campaign groups have emerged since the Health and Social Care Act was passed (Keep Our NHS Public; the NHS Support Federation; 38 Degrees…) and they have an abundance of information on their websites – there is even a new political party, the National Health Action Party. To echo some of the suggestions posed by these groups, on how to 'Save the NHS', here are some practical things that we can all consider doing to ensure it reaches Eighty:

Join an NHS campaign group to engage in discussions about local issues (such as hospital closures/cuts). The NHS Support Federation explains more about how to campaign: http://www.nhscampaign.org. uk/new_campaign_guide/fed_campaign_guide.html per cent232 Here is a list of some campaign groups:

A Better NHS https://abetternhs.net/about/ (Accessed May 2018)
Centre for Health and the Public Interest – Independent health think tank http://chpi.org.uk
Keep our NHS public – Campaigns for the NHS https:// keepournhspublic.com/ (accessed May 2018)
The NHS Support Federation – Pressure group that campaigns for the NHS http://www.nhscampaign.org
The National Health Action Party – Campaigns for the NHS https:// nhaparty.org
Patients4NHS – www.patients4nhs.org.uk
38 Degrees – online campaign organisation https://home.38degrees. org.uk
London Health Emergency – campaigns against NHS privatization since 1988 https://healthemergency.org.uk
NHS for Sale http://www.nhsforsale.info/

Engage with the NHS – by attending a local CCG board meeting, or a patient participation group at your GP surgery, and ask about members conflicts of interests. Challenge proposed changes to local services on anything other than clinical grounds and ask for a pro-NHS approach. There is a statutory requirement for NHS bodies to publicly consult when a significant change to the service is planned (such as hospital closures) and the NHS constitution gives us a right to be involved in the planning of healthcare services. Find out about local meetings (which are usually open to the public) by searching your local CCG, Trust or local authority webpage, or using your local Healthwatch: http://www.healthwatch.co.uk/find-local-healthwatch

Write to your MP and engage with local media. Find out who your MP is here: www.theyworkforyou.com and write a letter to your MP at The House of Commons, Westminster, London, SW1A0AA

Sources and Additional Reading

Books and articles

APPLEBY J, ABBASI K (2018) 'The NHS at 70: Loved, valued, affordable?' *BMJ* 361, 1540

BAIRSTOW, R. (2015) *The British Dentist*. Shire Library

BEGG N, RAMSAY M, WHITE J. (1998) 'Media dents confidence in MMR vaccine'. *BMJ* 316, 561

BEVAN, B., KARANIKOLOS,M., EXLEY, J., NOLTE, E., CONNOLLY, S. AND MAY, N. (2014) 'The four health systems of the United Kingdom: how do they compare?' Research report. The Nuffield Trust and Health Foundation

CARRIER E. (2013) 'High Physician Concern About Malpractice Risk Predicts More Aggressive Diagnostic Testing In Office Based Practice'. *Health Affairs* 32, 8, 383-1391

CRONIN, A.J. (1937) *The Citadel*. Pan Macmillan

DAVIS J, LISTER J, WRIGLEY D. (2015) *NHS for sale – Myths, lies and deception*. Merlin press.

DAVIS J, TALLIS R Ed. (2013) *NHS SOS - How the NHS was betrayed and how we can save it*. Oneworld

DAWSON, B. (1918) 'The future of the medical profession'. *Lancet*, 2, 83-85

DUCKWORTH, J. (2016) *Health and heartbreak - Healthcare before the NHS*. Austin Macauley Publishers Ltd

EL-GINGIHY Y (2015) *How to dismantle the NHS in 10 easy steps*. Zero Books

GODBER, G. (1988) 'Forty years of the NHS'. *BMJ*, 297, 37-43

GREEG, D. (2010) *Pauper Capital: London and the Poor Law 1790-1870*. Routledge, Aldershot

KMIETOWICZ, Z. (2006) *A century of general practice*. BMJ, 332, 7532, 39-40

LEWIS J, WILLIAMS A, FRANKLIN B, THOMAS J, MOSDELL N. (2008) *The Quality and Independence of British Journalism*. Cardiff: Cardiff University Media Department.

MCCARTNEY M. (2016) *The state of medicine – keeping the promise of the NHS*. Pinter & Martin

MCDERMOTT I, CHECKLAND K et al (2016) 'Engaging GPs in commissioning: realist evaluation of the early experiences of Clinical Commissioning Groups in the English NHS'. J Health Serv Res Policy, 22, 1, 4–11.

NASH L.M. (2010) 'Perceived practice change in Australian doctors as a result of medicolegal concerns'. *MJA* 193, 579-583

NIGHTINGALE, F. (1898) *Notes on Nursing What it is and What it is not*. D Appleton and Company, New York

PARKES, M & SHEARD, S. (2012) *Nursing in Liverpool since 1862*. Scotforth Books, Lancaster

PARKIN, E. (2017) The prescription charge and other NHS charges. House of Commons Library. Briefing Paper number 07227

PINDER, RJ. (2014) *The NHS in England An introduction for junior doctors*. Codex Project, London

POLLOCK, AM (2005) NHS Plc: *The Privatisation of our health care*. Verso Books

POLLOCK, AM (2016) *The End of the NHS*. Verso Books

RICHARDSON, R. (2013) 'A dismal prospect: Workhouse Healthcare'. *Lancet*, 382, 20-21

RIVETT, G. (1998) *From Cradle to Grave: Fifty years of the NHS*. King's Fund, London

RIVETT, GC (1986) *The development of the London hospital system 1823-1982*. London, King's Fund

ROBERTS, F. (1949) 'The cost of the NHS'. *BMJ*, 1, 293

ROGERS, J. (1889) *Reminiscences of a workhouse medical officer*. Fisher Unwin, London

SMITH, H.L. (2014) *Harry's last stand*. Icon Books Ltd

STUDDERT DM. (2005) 'Defensive Medicine Among High Risk Specialist Physicians in a Volatile Malpractice Environment'. *JAMA* 293, 21, 2609-2617

TAYLOR R. (2013) *God Bless the NHS-The truth behind the current crisis*. Faber & Faber guardianbooks

VAN BEKKUM JE, HILTON S. (2013) 'Primary care nurses' experiences of how the mass media influence frontline healthcare in the UK'. *BMC Fam Pract* 14, 178

WATSON, R. (1969) *Edwin Chadwick, Poor Law and Public Health*. Longman, Essex

WHITBY, L. (1948) 'The Changing Face of Medicine'. *BMJ*, 4565, 2-6

WHITFIELD, M. (2016) *The Dispensaries. Healthcare for the poor before the NHS. Britains forgotten health-care system.* AuthorHouse UK, Bloomington, USA

WILSON, N., GELBIER, S. (2014) *The Changes in Dentistry since 1948: The John McLean Archive – A Living History of Dentistry Witness Seminar 2.* British Dental Association

WOOLHANDLER S, HIMMELSTEIN DU (1997) 'Costs of care and administration at For-Profit and other hospitals in the United States'. *NEJM* 336, 769-774

Online sources

APPLEBY, J (2018) '70 years of NHS spending'. Nuffield Trust https://www.nuffieldtrust.org.uk/news-item/70-years-of-nhs-spending

Beveridge, W. (1942) Social Insurance and Allied Services (The Beveridge Report) available:

BMA (2018) Career break advice for GPs. https://www.bma.org.uk/advice/career/progress-your-career/career-break-gp-advice

CARR, H (2018) Why is there always a winter crisis in the NHS? Sky News https://news.sky.com/story/why-is-there-always-a-winter-crisis-in-the-nhs-11195502

DAVIES, M (2018) GP dilemma: A patient from overseas expects me to prescribe antibiotics. https://www.gponline.com/gp-dilemma-patient-overseas-expects-prescribe-antibiotics/article/1461364

Dentaid Charity website https://www.dentaid.org/uk/

Department of Health. (2015) The NHS Constitution. Williams Lee. Available here: https://www.gov.uk/government/publications/the-nhs-constitution-for-england (

Florence Nightingale museum website. http://www.florence-nightingale.co.uk

GMC https://www.gmc-uk.org

GP Induction and Refresher Scheme. GP National recruitment office. https://gprecruitment.hee.nhs.uk/induction-refresher

https://sourcebooks.fordham.edu/halsall/mod/1942beveridge.asp

https://www.bda.org/news-centre/press-releases/Pages/NHS-charges-masking-cuts-and-driving-patients-to-GPs.aspx

Kings Fund (2017) How the NHS is funded https://www.kingsfund.org.uk/projects/nhs-in-a-nutshell/how-nhs-funded

MATTHEWS-KING A. (2015) Hunt confirms rollback on pre-election pledge of 5000 new GPs. Pulse. http://www.pulsetoday.co.uk/news/new-deal-2015/16/hunt-   confirms-rollback-on-pre-election-pledge-of-5000-new-gps/20010348.fullarticle

MILLETT D. (2016) MPs Slam government 'complacency' over GP workforce crisis. GP Online. http://www.gponline.com/mps-slam-government-complacency-gp- workforce-crisis/article/1386541

Ministry of Health and Department of Health for Scotland. (1944) A National Health Service. London, HMSO. http://old.post-gazette.com/pg/pdf/201004/2010_national-health-service-book_01.pdf

MORAN V, ALLEN P et al. (2017) How are clinical commissioning groups managing conflicts of interest under primary care co-commissioning in England? A qualitative analysis http://bmjopen.bmj.com/content/7/11/e018422

MURPHY S (2018) NHS crisis? What crisis? http://www.dailymail.co.uk/news/article-5320623/NHS-doctors-ski-break-winter-emergency.html

National Health Service History http://www.nhshistory.net/

National life tables, UK: 2014-2016. (2017) Office for National Statistics. https://www.ons.gov.uk/peoplepopulationandcommunity/birthsdeathsandmarriages/lifeexpectancies/bulletins/nationallifetablesunitedkingdom/2014to2016

National Union of Journalists. (2011) NUJ Code of Conduct. Available: https://www.nuj.org.uk/about/nuj-code/

NAVARRO V (2003) 'The inhuman state of US Healthcare'. *Monthly Review*, 55, 4 https://monthlyreview.org/2003/09/01/the-inhuman-state-of-u-s-health-care

NHS Workforce Statistics, September 2017, Provisional Statistics https://digital.nhs.uk/catalogue/PUB30165

OCED. (2017) Health at a Glance 2017: OCED Indicators. OCED Publishing, Paris http://dx.doi.org/10.1787/health_glance-2017-en

Performer list policies and procedures. NHS England. https://www.england.nhs.uk/commissioning/primary-care/primary-care-comm/performer-list-policies-procedures/

TATTERSFIELD H (2013) GPs are already wise to the scam of new commissioning groups. The *Guardian* https://www.theguardian.com/commentisfree/2013/jan/21/gps-sham-ccgs-local-commissioning

Vaccinations – In 1948, children would be given smallpox and diphtheria vaccinations routinely. Today, the routine immunization schedule protects against 17 diseases (see here: https://www.gov.uk/government/uploads/system/uploads/attachment_data/file/633693/Complete_imm_schedule_2017.pdf for an up to date version of the routine immunization schedule

VAID N. (2010) 'Private sector providers in England: The implications of Independent sector treatment centres'. *Eurohealth*, 16, 3, 8-11 http://www.euro.who.int/__data/assets/pdf_file/0007/129436/Eurohealth16_3.pdf

WILLIAMS H, LEES C, BOYD M. (2014) the General Medical Council: fit to practice? Civitas Doctors Policy Research Group http://www.civitas.org.uk/pdf/GMCFittoPractise.pdf

Workhouses website. http://www.workhouses.org.uk

Index